MIDDLE EAR STRUCTURES

CONGENITA

MIDDLE EAR STRUCTURES, ORGANOGENESIS AND CONGENITAL DEFECTS

edited by
B. Ars and P. van Cauwenberge

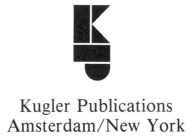

Kugler Publications
Amsterdam/New York

Library of Congress Cataloging-in-Publication Data

Middle ear structures, organogenesis, and congenital defects / edited
  by B. Ars and P. van Cauwenberge.
     p.   cm.
  "Made up of collected manuscripts from the symposium middle ear
structures, organogenesis, and congenital defects which took place
under the auspices of the Vth International Congress on Pediatric
Otology, held in Ghent, June 5–9, 1990" – Pref.
  Includes bibliographical references and index.
  ISBN 9062990746
  1. Middle ear – Differentiation – Congresses. 2. Middle ear –
–Histology – Congresses, 3. Middle ear – Abnormalities – Congresses.
I. Ars, B. II. Cauwenberge, P. van III. International Congress on
Pediatric Otology (5th : 1990 : Ghent, Belgium)
QP461.M65 1991
612.8′54 – dc20   91-12019
                                                                  CIP

ISBN 90-6299-074-6

Distributors:
For the U.S.A. and Canada:
Kugler Publications
P.O. Box 1498
New York, NY 10009-9998 USA
Telefax (+212) 477 1970

For Italy:
Ghedini Editore
Via della Signora, 6
20122 Milano – Italy
Telex 353113 GHEDI-I
Telefax (+39.2) 781150

For all other countries:
Kugler Publications bv
P.O. Box 516
1180 AM Amstelveen, The Netherlands
Telefax (+31.20) 6380524

Phototypeset by Palm Productions, Nieuwerkerk a/d IJssel, The Netherlands

CONTENTS

CONTENTS

Dedicated to Professor JEAN MARQUET

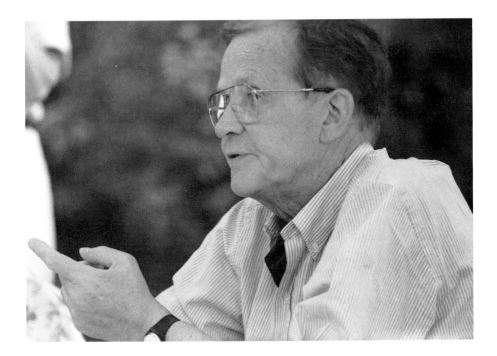

Pioneer in allograft tympanoplasty.

Exceptional otologist and oto-surgeon.
Admirable for his perceptiveness and touch,
he stirs up the whole concept and treatment of
congenital malformations of the middle ear.

PREFACE

This volume is made up of the collected manuscripts from the Symposium *Middle Ear Structures, Organogenesis and Congenital Defects* which took place under the auspices of the Vth International Congress on Pediatric Otology, held in Ghent, June 5–9, 1990.

The meeting provided the opportunity to bring together an international and multi-disciplinary group of experts, prominent authorities, working on the same subject matter.

Lecturers and topics are arranged as follows: The first papers deal with the more fundamental approaches to the organogenesis and structure of the middle ear. Then follow histology, histochemistry and physiology. The final part deals with new fundamental data leading to a more accurate clinical diagnosis and messages of experienced surgeons.

Apart from the research and explanation of definite details, the main theme has been the dynamics of organogenesis, the ulterior motive being the malleability of the different components and the role played by the interactions from one structure to the others.

The informality and intimacy of this meeting permitted discussion of current and incomplete research and stimulated lively speculations and arguments.

I would like to express my thanks to the many participants who attended the Symposium and particularly to the speakers who assisted in this publication by careful preparation of their papers.

I would also like to express my special appreciation to Professor Pol Van Cauwenberge, who gave me the opportunity to organize this Symposium.

Finally, I am most grateful to Kugler Publications of Amsterdam who made the publication of this book possible.

This book will have fulfilled its purpose if it succeeds in conveying to the reader the admiration felt by the participants for the captivating process of organogenesis of the structures of the middle ear.

BERNARD ARS

LIST OF CONTRIBUTORS

ARS, B.

Temporal Bone Foundation
68, avenue du Polo,
B-1150, Brussels, Belgium

ARS-PIRET, N.

Temporal Bone Foundation
68, avenue du Polo,
B-1150, Brussels, Belgium

DECLAU, F.

Department of Otorhinolaryngology
University of Antwerp,
Universiteitsplein, 1
B-2610, Wilrijk, Belgium

BERNAL-SPREKELSEN, M.

Department of Otorhinolaryngology
University of Bochum
St. Elisabeth Hospital
D-4630 Bochum, FRG

BOEDTS, D.

Department of Otorhinolaryngology
University of Antwerp,
Universiteitsplein, 1
B-2610, Wilrijk, Belgium

BROEKAERT, D.

Laboratory of Physiological Chemistry
State University of Ghent
K.L. Ledeganckstraat, 35
B-9000 Ghent, Belgium

FENART, R.

Laboratoire de Craniologie comparée
Faculté libre de Médecine
56, rue du Port
F-59046 Lille, France

JAHRSDOERFER, M.

Department of Otolaryngology,
Head and Neck Surgery
University of Texas Medical School
Houston, TX 77030, USA

MARQUET, J.

Department of Otorhinolaryngology
University of Antwerp
Universiteitsplein 1
B-2610, Wilrijk, Belgium

MICHAELS, L.   Department of Histopathology
                                         University College and Middlesex
                                         School of Medicine
                                         Institute of Laryngology and Otology
                                         330, Gray's Inn road
                                         London, WCLX 8EE, UK

SOUCEK, S.   ENT Audiology Department
                                         St Mary's Hospital
                                         Pread Street
                                         London, W2, UK

PHYLOGENIC CONSIDERATIONS ON THE MECANOMORPHOGENESIS OF THE MIDDLE EAR STRUCTURES

R. FENART
Directeur de Recherches au C.N.R.S., Laboratoire de Craniologie comparée, Faculté libre de Médecine, 56 Rue du Port, 59046 Lille Cédex, France

Introduction

The form of every element in the head of human beings is the result of progressive phenomena. They bring about mechanical interactions between classically known processes, particularly the encephalic development, upright posture and jaw reduction. This applies, among other things, to the ear ossicles[1].

The changes we will study in the ossicular chain, as well as those concerning the whole neurocranium and splanchnocranium, will be related to a common system of references: 'vestibular orientation'.[2, 3]

1. Methodology

In the vestibular method the organ (external semi-circular canal), is considered anatomically horizontal, just as, in the field of physiology, one looks at somebody's head from the left, the horizontal axis is defined (in a sagittal projection) as the general direction of this canal. The vertico-frontal axis is perpendicular, leading to the previous one and going through the middle of the canal buckle. The direction is considered in a positive way towards the top and back of the head. Thus each point will be exactly defined by its two coordinates (as width is not taken into account in this study).

Moreover, the diameter of the buckle of the semi-circular horizontal canal will be used here as a common measure of the dimensions of the ossicles and of the labyrinth, in order to be able to compare them directly with other species of mammals with quite a different size (ranging from a mouse of a few centimeters to a Sirenian of several meters !).

2. Equipment for study

The word 'phylogenesis' stands here for the study of adults from the present species compared with each other and *Homo sapiens*, in order to find the general 'laws', close to those that probably have governed the actual evolution, the stages of which are mostly only presumed.

However, how to start the investigation? First, we present Fig. 1 to the reader, which is certainly familiar to him, since it summarizes the Reichert-Gaupp classical theory[4]. But it is necesssary to note that a more recent theory has been proposed by Scandinavian paleontologists, according to investigations made on fossil Crossopterygian fishes. According to Jarvik and Stensiö[5], no change would occur in the nature of the bone operating in the mandibular articulation, and all the ear ossicles

Middle Ear Structure, Organogenesis and Congenital Defects, pp. 1–10
edited by B. Ars and P. van Cauwenberge
©*1991 Kugler Publications, Amsterdam, New York*

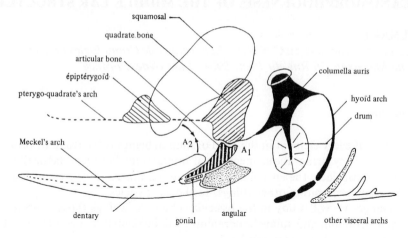

squamosal
quadrate bone
articular bone
épiptérygoïd
pterygo-quadrate's arch
columella auris
hyoïd arch
drum
Meckel's arch
A₂
A₁
dentary
gonial
angular
other visceral archs

REPTILIAN SPLANCHNOCRANIUM

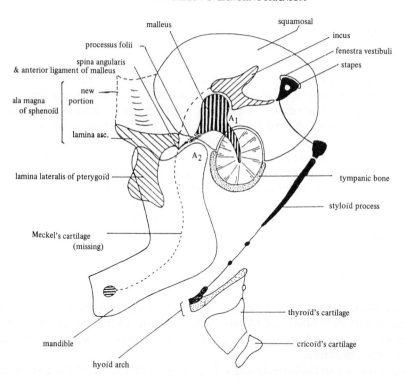

malleus
squamosal
incus
processus folii
fenestra vestibuli
spina angularis
& anterior ligament of malleus
stapes
new
portion
ala magna
of sphenoïd
A₁
lamina asc.
A₂
lamina lateralis of pterygoïd
tympanic bone
styloïd process
Meckel's cartilage
(missing)
thyroïd's cartilage
mandible
cricoïd's cartilage
hyoïd arch

MAMMALIAN SPLANCHNOCRANIUM

Fig. 1. Chief modifications of the ear region during the evolution: reptiles-mammals (classical theory).

would always have belonged to the hyoïdian arch (Fig. 2).

Our purpose is to study the bones which can be found in the middle ear, only for mammals, by taking into account the ossicles in their *proper place*, and not isolated from their anatomical environment.

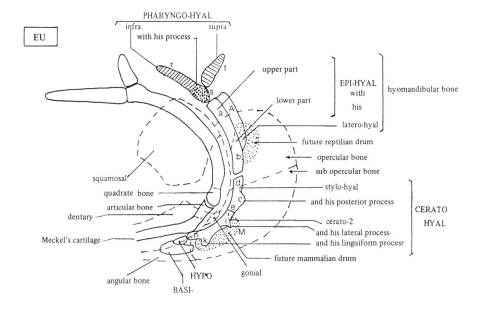

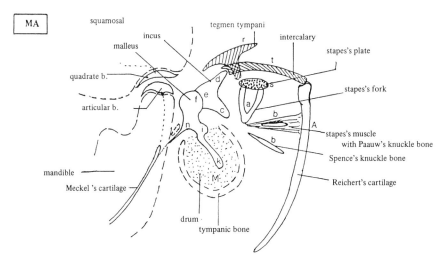

Fig. 2. Correspondence between elements of primitives archs, in a fossil fish (*Eusthenopteron*: Eu) and ossicular chain region in mammals (Ma), according to Jarvik[5].

Forty-one species have been used. They belong to all orders of the Mammifer class, ranging from Monotrems to human beings. Ossicles were immobilized with an injection of molten paraffin in the tympanic cavity, and the lateral semi-circular canal was visualized through dissection.

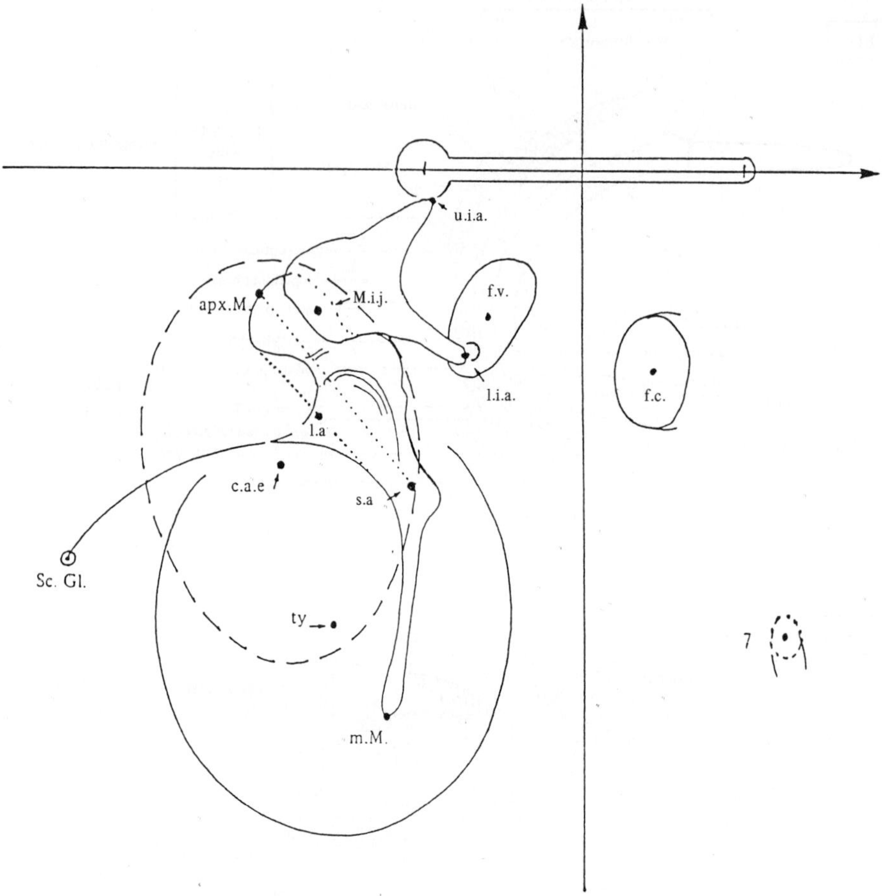

Fig. 3. Morphometric points used for systematization of the middle ear region (example with *Ovis aries*). The vestibular orientation is given by the two axes.

Apx.M.	= apex of the malleus head.
M.i.j.	= middle of malleo-incudal joint
s.a.	= short apophysis (processus lateralis)
l.a.	= long apophysis (processus folii)
m.M.	= lower part of the manubrium mallei
u.i.a.	= end of upper incudal apophysis
l.i.a.	= end of lower incudal apophysis, with lentiform bone.
f.v.	= center of the fenestra vestibuli
f.c.	= center of the fenestra cochleae

(see also Fenart[6]).

3. Interpretation

As to a statistical analysis, the interpretation of the results could have been facilitated by summarizing all the observations into five typical stages during which the main evolutive events occur: *Marsupials*, *non-Primate Eutherians*, *non-Anthropomorph Primates*, *Anthropomorphs*, and *Homo sapiens*. It is even possible to reduce them to four, by neglecting the simian primates.

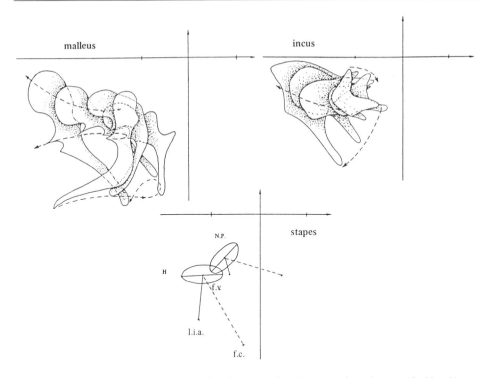

Fig. 4. Phylogenic evolution of the three ossicles in mammals. N.P. = quadruped mammals, H = Homo

On an ossicular chain and elements connected to it, 13 morphometric points have been defined (Fig. 3) and each of them has been positioned according to its two vestibular coordinates, after having drawn through to the common size of the horizontal canal diameter.

Under these conditions, as a result of statistical considerations which are not the purpose of this study (but which can be found in the first publication by G. Fenart[6]), it is possible to characterize the evolution of the mammalian ossicular chain by artificially isolating the three elements to clarify the iconography (Fig. 4).

There are considerable morphological changes especially as regard the malleus, but apart from this we can notice changes in the position of the three ossicles. The head of the malleus moves upwards clockwise in a circular way. Its long apophysis (processsus folii) advances and the lower part of the manubrium mallei moves backwards, then advances a little. The incus advances in a circular way, like the head of the malleus. The stapes undergoes, at its distal end, the fate of the lower apophysis of the incus, whereas its platin moves is the same way as the oval window does. The latter moves downwards and forwards in a circular way, whereas its great axis moves towards horizontality.

Let us add, as other investigations[7, 8] have shown, that the round window and the ampulla of the posterior semi-circular canal turn downwards in the same way and that the cochlea does so forwards and upwards. The conclusion is that in the mammalian labyrinth, if the direction of the external semi-circular canal is fixed horizontally, *all the other elements move* around the latter, so as to reproduce the phylogeni-

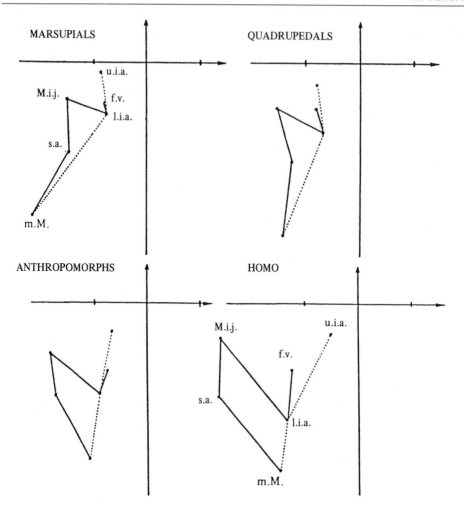

Fig. 5. Stylization of the ossicular chain, and (dotted) Helmoltz line.

cal rotative movement which can be seen in the posterior neurocranial portions. The same holds for the superior part of the ossicular chain. The movement towards a progressive straightening up of the body must be held responsible for this evolution.

On the other hand, it is the phylogenic backward movement of the jaws which can be felt on the manubrium mallei, thanks to the tympanic frame, and it manifests itself by a rotation of the manubrium mallei which is impressive because of its amplitude (near 120°).

Furthermore, taking into account noticeable morphometric points of the ossicles, it is possible to realize the huge changes on the segments used for the vibration transmission. By joining five points (Fig. 5) which schematically represent the whole chain, one can follow the morphological and positional evolution of the latter. The course which is represented by the broken line is becoming even longer and less direct, in spite of the fact that the end points are converging.

The anterior concavity of the malleus becomes a posterior concavity. In human

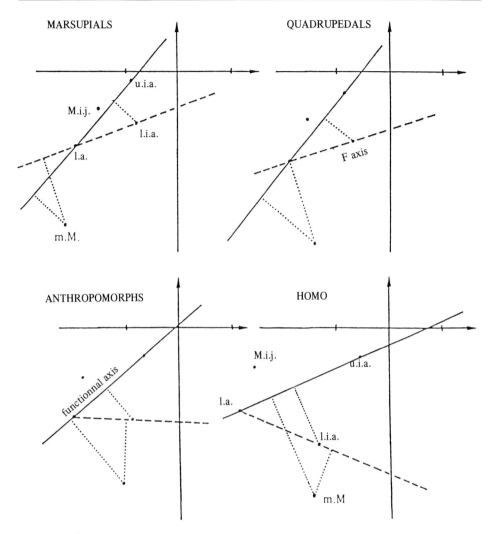

Fig. 6. Functional axis, after Dahmann (full line) and Fumagalli (axis F, dashed line).

beings the manubrium mallei has become parallel to the inferior branch of the incus and has obtained the same length. The posterior axis of the malleus head (s.a. – M.i.j.) has become equal and parallel to the transverse axis of the stapes (f.v. – l.i.a.).

The previous broken line has got two out of the three Helmoltz points[9]: m.M. and l.i.a., the third being u.i.a. (Fig. 5). The latter point turns in accordance with the two others and the alignment can only be achieved for Anthropomorphs (*cf.* Ardouin[10, 11]).

From the elements of Fig. 5 the *functional axis* can still be drawn, especially those of Dahmann[12] and Fumagalli[13] (Fig. 6). The Dahmann axis goes through l.a. and u.i.a. It turns by about 30° from lower mammals to *Homo sapiens*, in the same way as for the foramen magnum. The Fumagalli axis goes through l.a. and l.i.a. It turns in the same way as the previous one, but with a greater amplitude (43°).

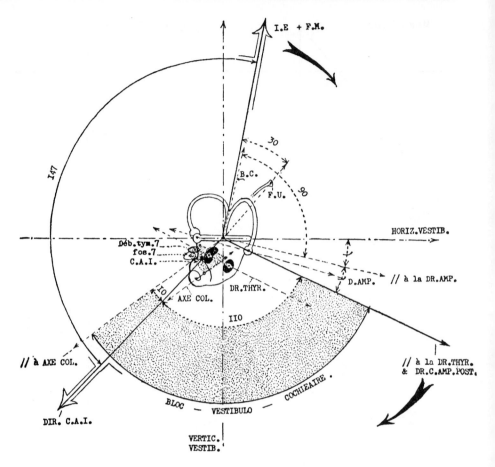

Fig. 7. Rotatory correlations between labyrinthine and cranial components, in quadruped mammals (for legend details, see Delattre[15].

The various 'lever arms' can be seen in the form of dotted lines in Fig. 6. Those by Dahmann are getting quite closer, especially through a backward movement of the most anterior one whose ends projected behind l.a. for Homo. Furthermore, they get longer in a differential way.

As for the lever arm of Fumagalli, its length decreases about by half, from the lower mammals to the human beings, and turns in the same way as the others.

4. Etiological implications

In addition to the backward movement of the manubrium mallei, which follows that of the jaws, one can see that the hominization of the ossicular chain is mainly linked with rotatory phenomena. Given the fact that this rotation exists not only in the labyrinth (the whole internal ear except the lateral semi-circular canal), but also on the back of the skull and on a part of the skull base, we were induced to study the rotatory amplitudes (Figs. 7 and 8).

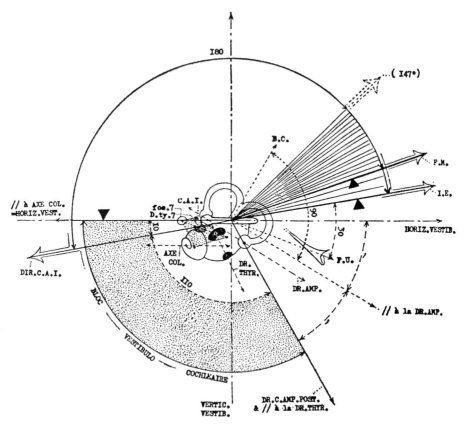

Fig. 8. As Fig. 7, in *Homo sapiens* (Delattre[15]). Please pay attention to overrotation drawn with fan-shaped lines.

Thus we can notice that the internal ear + the ossicles + the occipital bone + the base of the posterior skull, turn around the center of the horizontal semi-circular canal, with the same amplitude and homogeneity until the thyridian angle (between the straight line linking the center of the round and oval windows, and the horizontal canal) reaches 60°, *i.e.*, in the Australopithecides stage.

This occurs when a phylogenic stop of the rotation of the ear elements (including the oval window) happens while the bone elements, which are further from the rotatory axis (occipital bone, clivus . . .), *keep on turning* in the same way.

This 'overrotation' by 35° for the inion thus creates, in the human kind only, the appearance of a 'necessary but not sufficient condition' for the appearance of an otosclerosis, the other condition being the possible development of a histological disorder of the petrous bone. If these two factors are found together in a subject, the oval window is likely to be carried away from its maximum position through overrotation, flattening out the stapes platin.

Summarizing: The big evolutive processes which guide the morphogenesis of the head of *Homo sapiens* also appear in the labyrinth and in the ear ossicles. We must particularly underline the importance of the petro-occipital rotation, a phenomenon which comes along with the advent of the upward posture, a rotation which has a normal limit but which, in some circumstances in which this limit is surpassed, can held responsible for auditory disorders. This is the price to be paid for hominization.

References

1. Delattre A, Fenart R: Note sur les modifications ossiculaires chez les Mammifères. CR Ass Anat Toulouse 505–508, 1962
2. Delattre A, Fenart R: *L'Hominization du crâne étudiée par la méthode vestibulaire*, pp 418. Paris: CNRS 1960.
3. Girard L: Le plan des canaux semi-circulaires horizontaux considéré comme plan horizontal de la tête. Bull Soc Anthrop Paris 4: 14–33, 1923
4. Reichert C: Ueber die Visceralbögen der Wirbeltiere. Arch Anat Physiol 1837
5. Jarvik E: *Théories de l'évolution des vertébrés, reconsidérées à la lumière des récentes découvertes sur les vertébrés inférieurs.* Paris: Masson 1960
6. Fenart G: Etude vestibulaire de la chaîne ossiculaire des Mammifères. Problèmes étiologiques soulevés par son hominisation. Medical thesis. Lille 1982
7. Fenart R, Rousselle B: L'angle thyridien de l'homme adulte, sa variabilité. Bull Ass Anat Marseille 401–405, 1966
8. Saban R: Fixité du canal semi-circulaire externe et variations de l'angle thyridien. Mammalia XVI (2): 77–92, 1952
9. Helmoltz LF: Ueber die Mechanik der Gehörknöchelchen und des Trommelfells. Pflüg Arch Ges Physiol 1: 1–60, 1868
10. Ardouin P: Considérations anatomiques sur les osselets de l'ouïe chez certains singes anthropomorphes. Bull Soc Anthrop Paris 8 (5): 20–47, 1934
11. Ardouin P: Contribution à l'étude de la chaîne des osselets de l'ouïe chez les mammifères placentaires. Rev Laryngol (Paris) 62: 1–57, 121–130, 155–188, 214–265, 310–326, 1941
12. Dahmann H: Zur Physiologie des Hörens; experimentelle Untersuchungen ueber die Mechanik der Gehörknöchelchenkette, ueber deren Verhalten aus Ton und Luftdruck. Z Hals-Nasen-Ohrenheilk 24: 462–497, 1929
13. Fumagalli Z: Ricerche morfologiche sull'apparato di transmissione del suono. Arch Ital Otol-rhinol-laringol 60 (suppl.1): 1949
14. Delattre A, Fenart R: Evolution des fenêtres du vestibule, des mammifères à l'homme. Bull Soc Anthrop Paris II; XIth series 273–289, 1961
15. Delattre A, Fenart R: Formation des orifices de la face postérieure du rocher humain. Etude par la méthode vestibulaire au cours le la phylogénèse des mammifères et de l'ontogénèse humaine. Mammalia (Paris) 26 (2): 214–279, 1962

DYNAMICS OF THE ORGANOGENESIS OF THE MIDDLE EAR STRUCTURES
Anatomical variants

BERNARD ARS and NICOLE ARS-PIRET

Temporal Bone Foundation, Avenue du Polo, 68, B-1150 Brussels, Belgium

Introduction

As a result of the assembling of quite a number of constituent structures, the middle ear presents an eminently complex morphology. It constitutes an integration of several embryonic tissues and is composed of the three fundamental embryological tissue layers.

The purpose of this study is to bring to the fore the *Dynamics* of the construction of this intricated puzzle, pointing out some anatomical particularities of the middle ear we note as more or less severe *modifications* of the *normal* morphology.

They are *particularities* or *variants* which are not considered to be anomalies or pathologic phenomena because of the frequency of their occurrence. Nevertheless, their presence and incidence require explanation.

These variants are tiny morphological modifications, surgical observations which may sometimes be correlated with certain clinical or functional events.

First, we briefly recapitulate the normal development of each constitutive structure of the middle ear, with emphasis on the most important key stages, and then consider the three-dimensional organization of those elements, in their individual development and at the same time in the general development of the middle ear, of the temporal bone and also of the skull. Then we will give some examples of the most common anatomical variants, and discuss them taking into account time sequences such as growth interactions.

I. Embryology of the constitutive structures of the middle ear

The middle ear is an irregularly shaped cavity, air-filled, situated in the heart of the temporal bone. It is made up of the tympanic, squamous, and petrous parts of the temporal bone which articulates with the occipital, parietal, sphenoid, and zygomatic bones. The whole of it contributes to the lateral wall and base of the skull and forms part of the middle and posterior cranial fossae. The middle ear opens anteriorly into the Eustachian tube and posteriorly into the tympanic antrum and mastoid air cells.

The ossicular chain is suspended into the middle ear cavity connecting the tympanic membrane with the oval window.

We surely do not intend to explain in detail the morphology of each constituent structure of the middle ear. For this, we refer to the outstanding publications of Bast and Anson[1,2].

However, the understanding of the variants of the middle ear is based on the

Middle Ear Structure, Organogenesis and Congenital Defects, pp. 11–25
edited by B. Ars and P. van Cauwenberge
©*1991 Kugler Publications, Amsterdam, New York*

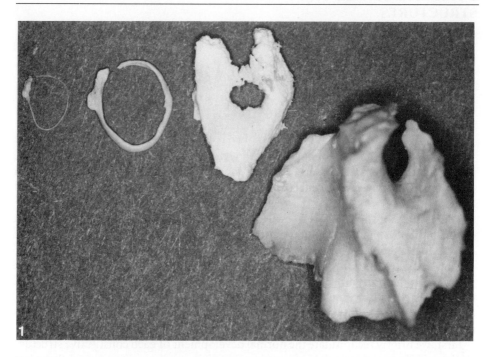

Fig. 1. The tympanic part of the temporal bone has been isolated to illustrate the most important stages of the development. 1a: Tympanic ring in an 11-week-old embryo. 1b: The tympanic ring increases in overall size: 19-week-old embryo. 1c: Tympanic bone of a five-month-old child: growth of the two tympanic tubercles which delimit the foramen of Huschke. 1d: Tympanic bone isolated from the temporal bone of a three-year-old child. Definite size and shape.

knowledge of the embryologic events. We intend to report briefly the most important stages of their organogenesis.

In the course of the development of the middle ear, the fundamental components are: the tympanic bone and membrane, the ossicular chain, the squamous bone, the petrous bone.

1. Tympanic bone and membrane

The development of the tympanic bone and membrane is already clearly defined as early as the fourth week of intra-uterine life[3].

A funnel-shaped ectoblastic pouch grows inwards from the first branchial cleft until it reaches a similar pouch growing laterally from the first endoblastic cleft, the tubo-tympanic recess. The contact between these two epithelial pouches is short-lived and lost temporarily because, as early as in the sixth week, the mesenchyme interposes as the head grows.

At the eighth week the epithelial cells at the bottom of the ectoblastic pouch proliferate and form a compact epithelial plate reaching the endoblast. This ectoblastic plate dissolves and the epithelial wall at the bottom of the pouch participates in the formation of the fibrous layer of the lamina propria of the tympanic membrane.

The first of the four small ossification centers of the membrane bone of the tym-

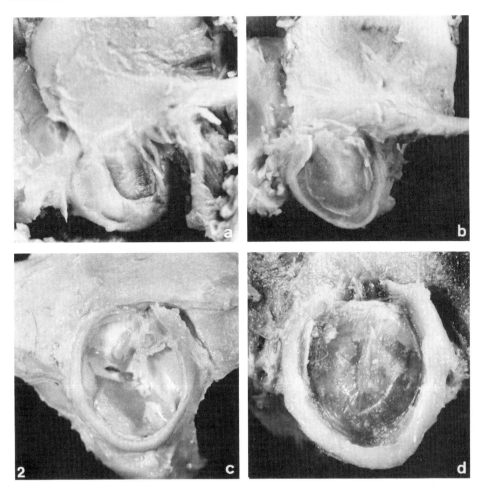

Fig. 2. a: Lateral view of the right temporal bone of a 12-week-embryo. The tympanic ring is formed; the half circle is open upward and backward. b: Right temporal bone of a 15-week-embryo. c: Tympanic bone *in situ* in a 19-week-embryo. d: The similar structure in a 35-week-old fetus.

panic ring appears at approximately nine weeks. The fusion of the four centers occurs at 11 weeks (Fig. 1a).

The bony tympanic ring is formed at the periphery of the tympanic membrane, the margin of which becomes inserted into the tympanic sulcus[4].

At 12 weeks, growth proceeds rapidly with a consequent increase in overall size (Fig. 2a).

The tympanic ring is almost fully developed by the 16th week (Fig. 2b).

The tympanic membrane appears already with its three layers; it has the form of an ellipse approximately 2 mm in horizontal diameter. It is clearly tightly set in a groove forming nine-tenths of a circle and extends upwards into the future epitympanum. After the 19th week of fetal life, the shape of the tympanic membrane does not change any more (Fig. 2c).

The tympanic bone is still independent of the otic capsule. Its fusion with the other

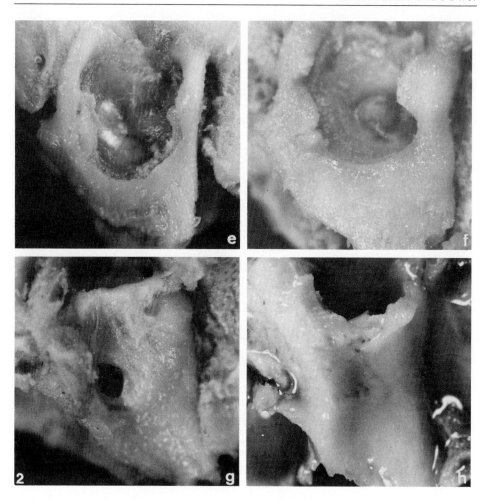

Fig. 2. e: Right tympanic part of a newborn. f: four-month-old child. g: 6½-month-old child. h: two-year-old child.

components of the temporal bone begins not until the age of 31 weeks in the posterior part. The antero-medial segment does not join until 40 weeks. (Fig. 1b and 2d).

Fixation is complete in the newborn. At birth (Fig. 2e), the tympanic bone still has the shape of a ring, broken at the top, the hiatus being the incisure of Rivinius. The diameter is 9 mm, *i.e.*, almost the definitive size[5-8].

After birth the tympanic bone grows in two directions (Fig. 1c,d, and 2f,g,h). Its medial side develops medially and comes into contact with the petrous bone. It becomes attached to the latter and participates in the formation of the lateral wall of the tympanic cavity. Its extension results from the growth of two tympanic tubercles which merge to delimit two openings: The first, in the upper part, is the new tympanic frame. The second, more lateral and below, is the foramen of Huschke which normally closes, like a diaphragm, before the age of five years[9].

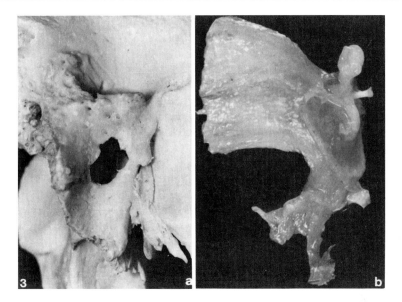

Fig. 3. a: Right tympanic part of a 12-year-old child. Temporal surface showing a persisting foramen of Huschke. b: Tympano-ossicular system. A skin invagination grew into a persisting foramen of Huschke in a 54-year-old man.

This foramen may however persist in a few rare cases: in 300 adult temporal bones we observed two cases of persisting foramen of Huschke (Fig. 3a). In both cases, the skin of the external auditory canal invaginated into the opening and under the inferior wall of the canal (Fig. 3b).

Huschke was the famous otologist who gave his name to this foramen, recording in details, in 1832, the outstanding observations of Duverney (1679)[10].

The overall growth of the tympanic bone contributes largely to the wall of the mandibular fossa, non-articular portion, and covers the styloid process anteriorly. It forms the anterior and inferior walls and a part of the posterior wall of the external auditory canal. Its development lateralwards leaves the tympanic sulcus and therefore the tympanic membrane insertions nearer to the midline.

2. Ossicular chain

We surely do not intend to solve the riddle of the origin of the ossicles. The subject has been a controversial one and there have been almost as many opinions as investigators. The consensus now is that the ossicles have multiple origins.

The ossicles are derived from the mesenchyme of the first and second branchial arches. The head and neck of the malleus, and the body of the incus differentiate from the first arch (mandibular visceral bar), while the second arch (hyoid visceral bar) gives rise to the manubrium of the malleus, the long proces of the incus and the superstructure of the stapes.

The greater part is first formed as cartilage models. The anterior process of the malleus, however, emerges from intramembranous ossification distinct from the visceral bars.

The stapes footplate has also a dual origin, partly from the second arch and partly from the otic capsule.

The ossicles are first seen in the four-week-old fetus. They are little areas of condensation of mesenchyme appearing as bridges connecting the two visceral arches. They grow rapidly in size. During the sixth week, precartilage forms in the future ossicles. Rapid transformation into true cartilage occurs during the seventh week.

By the end of the eighth week, the general configuration of the cartilaginous malleus closely approximates that of the adult. After that, a progressive and prodigious ossicular growth occurs and, by the 20th week, the ossicles are of adult size and begin to ossify.

The ossification of the incus takes place slightly earlier than that of the malleus, and in the 25- to 26-week-old fetus both incus and malleus are fully ossified with the exception of the distal extremity of the handle of the malleus. They achieve adult size and shape before birth. Likewise, the middle ear muscles and blood supply are fully developed at term.

3. The squamous bone

In the same way as the tympanic part, the squamous part of the temporal bone develops from a membrane. The squamous bone is formed from a center of ossification which appears in the eighth week.

The development differs for the upper and the lower halves of the membrane: The upper part is flat and thin. It will become the vertical portion. Its inferior margin continues with the lower or inferior part.

By the 16th week, because of the impediment formed by the presence of the tympanic bone, the inferior part of the membrane bulges and grows rapidly into three directions:

The anterior portion turns round forward and becomes fixed to the anterosuperior part of the tympanic bone. The middle part sinks medially to define the anterior wall of the epitympanic cavity and to contribute to the lateral wall of the tympanic cavity. The posterior part extends posteriorly to the tympanic ring forming the anterior portion of the mastoid process[11].

The postnatal growth of the squamous bone is due to the outward displacement by the enlarging skull. The squamous portion participates in the formation of the roof of the temporo-mandibular joint, anteriorly, it lines great part of the base of the petrous bone, posteriorly, and, through the middle part, it forms the superior wall of the external auditory canal and the external half of the epitympanum.

4. The petrous bone

The petrous portion is derived from the otic capsule and preformed in cartilage. Ossification of the cartilaginous model proceeds rapidly, originating from 14 centers appearing at approximately 16 weeks. By the 20th week, all centers have fused to form a complete bony capsule. Ossification is completed only shortly before birth.

The petrous bone constitutes a three-sided pyramid widely hollowed to harbor the membranous labyrinth, the semicircular canals and many fossae and canals transmitting blood vessels and nerves, the detailed description of which is outside the scope of our subject here (see refs.[1,2,4]).

The base of the pyramid forms the medial wall of the tympanic cavity. The major feature of this wall is the promontorium produced by the bulging basal turn of the cochlea and the two accompanying niches.

The oval window niche situated posteriorly and superiorly to the promontorium, harbors the stapes. It is limited superiorly by the facial nerve. Lower, the round window niche and its occluding round window membrane is located in the postero-inferior part of the medial wall. It is delimitated antero-superiorly by the promontorium and inferiorly by the hypotympanum.

Within the petrous bone, the so-called apical air cells occur in widely varying extent, appearance, size, number and distribution. They are pneumatic spaces which develop in a manner similar to that which produces the cavities of the tympanic cavity (see section II 3, *Pneumatization of the middle ear*).

II. Organogenesis of the tympanic cavity and of the middle ear

The static analysis of each constituent structure of the middle ear is used, in fact, to present the actors. The play itself requires a dynamic approach.

We will consider now, successively, the formation of the tympanic cavity, the antrum and mastoid process; the pneumatization and segmentation of the middle ear, and in the same way, we will observe the verticalization of the plane of the middle ear cavity as well as the accompanying evolution of the curvature of the tympanic membrane.

1. Formation of the tympanic cavity

The tympanic cavity and the lining of the middle ear and of the Eustachian tube are endodermal. They are originating from the first pharyngeal pouch which grows laterally, at about four weeks, and expands rapidly to pre-form two fundamental structures; (1) the distal part forms the tubotympanic recess, the future primitive tympanic cavity[3]; (2) the proximal part constricts to form the Eustachian tube.

The primitive tympanic cavity gradually expands like a growing bud and includes the ossicles and their associated muscles and blood vessels. The accompanying dissolution of the mesenchyme facilitates this progression.

Starting in the inferior half of the future middle ear, the extension of the cavity becomes thwarted upstairs by a projection of the otic capsule: the superior periotic process, which will constitute the superior wall of the middle ear, and downstairs by the bony wall of the floor of the middle ear originating from independent bone or from a lamellar projection of the petrous pyramid. The possible progression goes on in the sagittal plane giving rise, only late in fetal life, to the epitympanic recesses, the antrum and the mastoid air cells.

The tympanic cavity has virtually completed its expansion at about 33 weeks. The epitympanum follows approximately four weeks later.

2. Formation of the antrum and mastoid process

As a result of the fusion of the periosteal layers of the otic capsule and the tympanic process of the squamous bone, the mastoid process begins to develop at about 29 weeks.

A posteriorly directed evagination of the epitympanum begins the formation of the antrum which is well developed by the 35th week. As early as this period cavitation extends into the mastoid.

At 34 weeks, the pneumatization of the *mastoid* may really only just start, and progresses during infancy and childhood. As the mastoid grows, the antrum shrinks in relative size and assumes a more medial position. When the antrum is well formed and situated, the ventrolateral wall continues to grow until puberty or beyond that period, to give rise to the bone of the mastoid.

3. Pneumatization of the middle ear

The origin of the pneumatized spaces of the tympanic cavity, associated spaces and mastoid is tightly fixed.

During the first 12 weeks of fetal life, the cartilaginous cells, precursors of the ossicles, are embedded in a loose mesenchyme which limits the expansion of the future *tympanic cavity*. The epithelium from the auditory tube invades it. It divides into four sacci expanding into four different directions, lining the tympanic cavity with epithelium and enveloping the ossicles[12,13].

– The saccus anticus extending into the cranio-frontal direction will form the anterior pouch of von Trölsh.

– The saccus medius forms the attic; it extends upward and usually breaks into three smaller saccules.

– The saccus superior extends posteriorly and laterally between the malleus handle and the long crus of the incus; it forms the posterior pouch of von Trölsh.

– The saccus posterior extends along the hypotympanum to form the round window niche, sinus tympani and oval window niche.

These sacci are very important because they are at the origin of the segmentation of the middle ear.

Pneumatization of the tympanum is followed by that of the *associated air spaces*.

The antrum, a lateral extension of the epitympanum begins to form at about the age of 22 weeks. The mastoid and the antral air cells develop as an outgrowth of the antrum.

Epithelial buds from the middle ear spaces and antrum extend to adjacent areas of the temporal bone, after osteoclastic resorption of bone or differentiation of bone marrow into loose mesenchyme.

Thus, mastoid buds from the antrum penetrate to give rise to the mastoid air cells. The degree of pneumatization of the mastoid varies greatly in normal temporal bones. The distinction between 'pneumatic' and 'apneumatic' mastoid distinguishes the specimens in which the air cells are extensively developed from those with a mere indication of formation of air cells.

The age at which the air cells develop is subject to considerable individual variation. In contrast to the labyrinth and middle ear, the mastoid shows postnatal growth in length, width and depth[14].

4. Segmentation of the middle ear

As the tympanic cavity expands to include the ossicles, its epithelium covers the walls in the same way as the ossicles. Where two sacci oppose each other, a mucosal fold is formed and acts as a mesentery containing blood vessels.

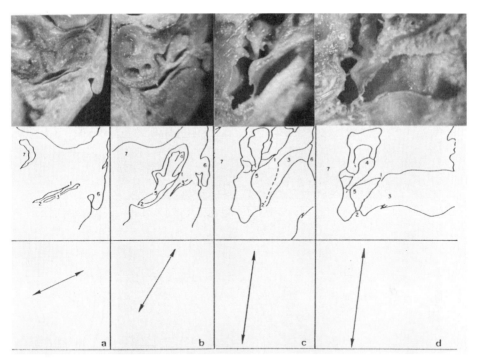

Fig. 4. Frontal section through the right external auditory meatus. a: The tympanic cavity and the internal auditory meatus of a 12-week-old fetus. (1) superior edge of the tympanic membrane, (2) inferior edge of the tympanic membrane, (3) external auditory meatus, (4) head of the malleus, (5) tympanic membrane, (6) auricle, (7) inner ear. b: The same section in a 19-week-old fetus: The caudal middle portion of the tympanic membrane is pushed laterally and the tympanic part comes gradually nearer the vertical. c: The same section in a four-month-old child. The tympanic membrane verticalizes, the tympanic cavity becomes noticeably larger. d: The same section in a three-year-old child. The shape and relationships of the tympanic bone and cavity are roughly the same as in the adult.

In this process the middle ear structures become ensheathed in a lining mucous membrane similar to the development of the abdominal visceral peritoneum. This mucous membrane divides into mucosal folds which carry blood vessels to the ossicles and, at the same time, divide the middle ear into several definite compartments.

Remarkable studies of Eden[15] suggest the presence of a visceral regulatory mechanism in which the brainstem both monitors and regulates the degree of the middle ear aeration.

5. Verticalization of the plane of the middle ear cavity

The development of the tympanic membrane follows that of the temporal bone and particularly its tympanic part. Emphasis is placed on the fact that the development of the tympanic part laterally leaves the tympanic sulcus, and therefore the eardrum insertions, nearer to the midline. Considerable changes occur in the orientation of the plane together with those morphological developments. These are consequent to the whole temporal bone development[16].

This is clearly demonstrated in frontal sections passing through the external auditory meatus, the tympanic cavity and the inner ear (Fig. 4).

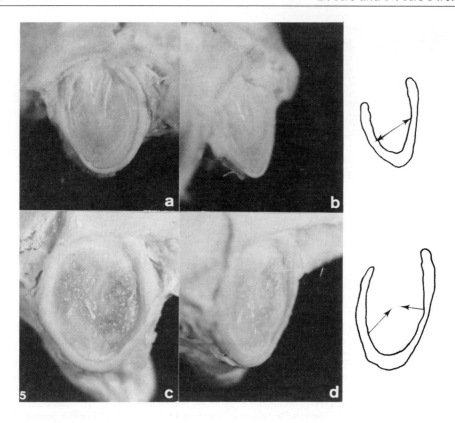

Fig. 5. Curvature of the tympanic membrane: a: External view of a 15-week-old embryo. b: The same piece in profile: the tympanic membrane appears flat. c: External view of a 31-week-old embryo. d: The same piece in profile: the concavity grows progressively.

At the age of 12 weeks of intrauterine life the tympanic part lies superficially and almost horizontally, situated in a plane oriented slightly obliquely, downward and medially (Figs. 2a and 4a). The tympanic part has the shape of a crescent opening upwards and backwards. The upper, or cranial end of this crescent is located in front of the malleus and laterally to its anterior process (Fig. 2b).

During growth, the squamous temporal bone moves laterally away from the midline, increasing the transverse diameter of the cranial cavity. In the course of this growth, the tympanic frame is pushed laterally so that its plane becomes vertical and its inferior surface becomes more lateral; it has the developing tympanic membrane within it.

During the 19th week of intrauterine life, the diameter of the tympanic part of the temporal bone increases by a half, to form nine-tenths of a circle (Figs. 2c and 4b). After this period, the shape of this tympanic part will remain virtually unchanged.

At 31 weeks, the tympanic cavity becomes quite large. The plane of the tympanic part of the temporal bone is then pushed laterally.

Four months after birth, the lateral movement continues and the orientation of the tympanic part becomes more or less the same as that of the adult (Fig. 4c).

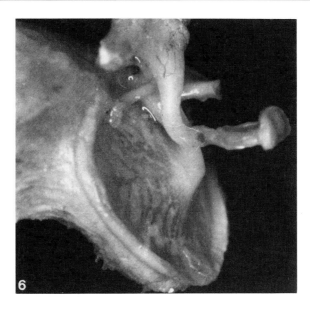

Fig. 6. Tympano-ossicular system of a 27-year-old man. From this view we observe the convexity of the tympanic membrane of the adult.

In a three-year-old child, the morphology and the spatial orientation of the tympanic part of the temporal bone are identical to those of an adult (Fig. 4d).

6. Evolution of the curvature of the tympanic membrane

The curvature of the tympanic membrane also depends on the age of the fetus (Fig. 5). At the 15th week of intra-uterine life, the eardrum is plane, flat (Fig. 5a,b). The concavity grows progressively with age. The concave shape of the tympanic membrane is a result of the suspension device of the ossicles within the middle ear. The long process of the malleus tends to retract the tympanic membrane into the middle ear cavity.

For example, the distance between the umbo and the annulus plane of a 31-week-old fetus is 0.9 mm (Fig. 5c,d). Further, in an 11-month old child, the distance between umbo and the annulus plane is 1.6 mm. In the adult, the equivalent distance is 2.1 mm. (Fig. 6)[17].

III. Some anatomical variants of the normal anatomy of the middle ear

Because it is not possible to report here all the variants observed, even less all the modifications stemming from a particularly intricated organogenesis, we have chosen to propose some examples as representative illustrations.

The fusion of the two arms of the tympanic bone, with the other components of the temporal bone, takes place during a relatively long period of time. The definitive coupling, more or less rapid, is responsible for minute particularities in the normal morphological development.

Ninety-one percent of the external auditory canals we have to dissect out for tympanoplasty, because of chronic otitis media, show protruding lateral posterior bony cristae[18].

In the same way, considering the tympanic bone and the otic capsule as two reference points during organogenesis, these also remain morphological landmarks in the adult.

In 300 normal adult temporal bones we have studied[8], the variations of the tympanic membrane and its lining sulcus project onto the medial wall of the tympanic cavity.

The projection of the tympanic sulcus totally overlapped the oval window in 9% of the cases. It overlapped the posterior two-thirds of the oval window in 34% of the cases. It overlapped the posterior third of the oval window in 48%. There was no overlap in 9% of the cases.

The same observation concerning the round window shows the following facts: The projection of the tympanic sulcus totally overlapped the round window in 31% of the cases; it overlapped the lower three-fourths in 11% of the cases; in 35.5% it overlapped the lower half, and in 22.5% the round window was completely visible.

These observations are the result of analysis of morphological plane projections.

A tri-dimensional point of view is illustred in the following observations:

The first concerns the spatial orientation of the external auditory canal and the tympanic cavity. The criteria are: the shape of the isthmus, the angle between the roof of the canal and the tympanic membrane, the form of the pretympanic sinus[19].

We have found a crucial relationship between these elements: a deep pretympanic sinus is always associated with a larger angle, more than 135°; when the sinus is absent, the angle is reduced, less than 125°.

The depth of the tympanic cavity is not a constant value. From the malleus inserted into the tympanic membrane, on the one hand, to the stapes confined into the oval window, on the other hand, the organization of the whole ossicular chain has to be adapted consequently.

Discussion

When we reported the most important steps of the peculiar organogenesis of the fundamental components of the middle ear, we intended to illustrate that each piece of the temporal bone constitutes a part of a *living puzzle*, which has to grow for itself, and at the same time, fuse with the other also growing elements, immersed in unstable surroundings.

If there is just a minute delay or a tiny modification in the sequence of these programmed events, we note more or less severe *modifications* of the *normal morphology*. Every embryological event occurs closely linked, intricated and intermingled, with those involving the neighboring structures. It may at the same time be the originator of a whole series of oncoming modifications.

The effects of the modifications are not always so evident and expressive as, for example, the well-known chain of disturbances in differentiation of the first pharyngeal pouch which will affect the architecture of the Eustachian tube and middle ear cavity, as well as the extent and character of the pneumatization of the tympanic cavity antrum and mastoid process. Nevertheless, discussing here only normal morphology and not pathology, the examples of morphological variants previously pointed to seem to be not very important in themselves, being only particularities. They should only be mentioned in well-specialized books on morphology if they could be just one link in the chain and sometimes lead to subsequent repercussions on the other morphological elements.

As to the tympanic bone, its development and fusion with the other components of the temporal bone: we integrate in a dynamic manner the variants observed, and believe that the displacement of the landmarks in relation with each other during embryogenesis and growth are manifestations of the same fact: a slight rotational shifting of the tympanic ring during its early development or, more precisely, a lack of coordination in the uncoiling of the tympanic ring with the other pieces constituting the temporal bone. This could be the cause of an arm of the tympanic bone protruding into the external auditory canal.

Moreover, we observed a kind of more or less discreet sagittal sliding of the plane of the tympanic bone in relation with the plane of the promontorium. Antero-posterior shifting leads to more or less overlapping of the round or the oval window. The moment of anchoring of the arms of the tympanic bone, being different for the anterior arm and for the posterior arm, could give rise to a sagittal sliding of the tympanic ring and, later on, of the tympanic sulcus.

Thus, one may wonder about the accompanying structures such as the three layers of the future tympanic membrane which would be inserted into the tympanic sulcus.

We touch here on the problem of the origin of the retraction pockets and cholesteatoma[20]. A further reflection on the appreciation of the torsion movements is that the most frequent types of retraction pockets involve anteriorly the pars flaccida or posteriorly the pars tensa. The rotation epicenter would be localized in the epitympanum.

What about the accompanying torsions and tractions of the mucosal folds in the tympanic cavity and the consequences on drainage and ventilation of the tympanic cavity, and what about the resulting disturbances of nerve and blood supply and their well-known action on the local metabolism?

Wullstein[21] still emphasized the role played by the mucosal lining in the health of the tympanic cavity. The mucosal folds build different floors of air cushions, considered as protections, as damping system for absorption of the overloading energy. On the other hand, Marquet[22] suggests the presence of an antro-tympanal interface playing a main role in the progression of middle ear infections.

The folds, together with the ligamentous tissues and ossicles constitute a real barrier which divides the middle ear cleft into two separated gas pockets: a posterior one, antro-mastoid cavity, considered as a truly open non-ventilated gas pocket and the anterior one, the tympanum, an open, intermittently ventilated gas pocket.

Both the lining mucous membrane and mucosal folds intervene in the aerodynamics of the middle ear cleft. Variations in position, orientation or extension could be the cause of severe disorders.

We know, according to Lim[23], that the smallest change in the mucous membrane lining may interfere with proper ventilation of the tympanic cavity. Marquet demonstrated that a part of the mucosa is covered with cilia which appear related to the clearance function of the middle ear. Qualitative or quantitative changes in this function could be heavily influencing the future tympanic cavity.

According to the histological point of view, another important factor in the relative time and spatial organization is the following: we know that a sufficient amount of mesenchyme is essential for the growth of migrating epidermal buds[24]. More or less rapid resorption of the mesenchyme of the branchial arch junction may result in the loss of the growth support for the epidermoid migration and consequently in lowering of the tissue guidance.

We would like to consider some observations or associations:

– The outstanding spine tympanica is more often associated with cholesteatoma[20].

– The torsion or traction of the pars tensa and of the folds after gentle displacement of the tympanic bone and the frequency of the retraction pockets.

– The change in orientation of the plane of the tympanic membrane and the associated altered orientation of the manubrium and ossicular chain.

– The tight relationship between the depth of the pretympanic sinus and the angle between the roof of the auditory canal and the tympanic membrane.

– The importance of a well-pneumatized mastoid: Sadé and Hadas[25] mentioned that the prognosis of chronic otitis media is related to the size of the mastoid air cells. The degree of mastoid pneumatization is an important prognostic sign of the clinical course of this pathology.

According to the position of the walls, the shape, size, connections and relationship to each other and their surrounding structures, the middle ear shows a wide range of variability.

Our attention has been directed to the construction and contents of the middle ear, to the embryologic origin as well as to the clinical and surgical significance of the variants of the structures observed.

A discussion of practical considerations has been included to correlate the anatomic details with their applications to clinical problems.

References

1. Bast Th, Anson S: *The Temporal Bone and the Ear*. Springfield (IL): CC Thomas Publications 1947
2. Anson B, Donalson J: *The Surgical Anatomy of the Temporal Bone and Ear*, pp. 492. Philadelphia, London, Toronto: WB Saunders Co 1973
3. Langman J: *Embryologie médicale*, pp 344. Paris: Masson 1965
4. Anson B, Bast Th, Richany S: The fetal early postnatal development of the tympanic ring and related structures in man. Ann Oto-Rhino-Laryngol 64: 802–823, 1955
5. Ars B, Decraemer W, Marquet J, Ars-Piret N: Sulcus tympanicus. In: Comptes-rendus du Congrès de la Société Française d'ORL, pp 401–468. Paris: Arnette 1980
6. Ars B, Ars-Piret N: Mouvements embryogéniques de l'anneau tympanique. In: Comptes-rendus du Congrès de la Société Française d'ORL, pp 117–119, Paris: Arnette 1981
7. Ars B: *Pars Tympanica Ossis Temporalis*. Academical thesis, *d'agregation de l'Enseignement superieur*. University of Antwerp 1982
8. Ars B: La partie tympanale de l'os temporal. Cahiers ORL 18: 435–523, 1983
9. Ars B: Foramen of Huschke. Valsalva, 60(3): 205–211, 1984
10. Duverney G: *Trait de l'Organe de l'Ouie*. 1683. Reedition Leyden, J Langerak (ed) 1931
11. Schuknecht H: *Pathology of the Ear*, pp 503. Cambridge (MA): Harvard University Press 1974
12. Proctor B: The development of the middle ear spaces and their surgical significance. J Laryngol Otol 78(7): 630–649, 1964
13. Marquet J: Congenital middle ear malformations. Acta Oto-Rhino-Laryngol Belg 42(2): 149–170, 1988

14. Eby Th, Nadol J: Postnatal growth of the human temporal bone. Implications for cochlear implants in children. Ann Otol Rhinol Laryngol 95: 356–364, 1986
15. Eden A: Neural control of middle ear aeration. Arch Otolaryngol Head Neck Surg 113: 133–137, 1987
16. Ars B, Ars-Piret N: The morphogenesis of the tympanic part of the temporal bone. Clin Otolaryngol 11: 9–13, 1986
17. Ars B, Ars-Piret N, Decraemer W: Design of the most natural middle ear device. In: *Transplants and Implants in Otology*, Proc International Symp, 6–9 April 1987, Venice, Italy, pp 27–34. Amsterdam, Berkeley, Milano: Kugler and Ghedini Publ 1988
18. Ars B, Decraemer W, Ars-Piret N: Lamina propria et rétractions tympaniques. Details morphologiques et physiques. Cahiers ORL 21(4): 283–289, 1986
19. Ars B: Allogreffes tympano-ossiculaires. Techniques chirurgicales. Morphologie et physiologie. Arq Portugueses Otorrinolaringol Patol Cervico-Facial 6(3 and 4): 5–23, 1987
20. Ars B, Decraemer W: Tympanic membrane lamina propria and middle ear cholesteatoma. In: Proc Third International Conference on Cholesteatoma and Mastoid Surgery, 5–9 June 1988, Copenhagen. Amsterdam, Berkeley, Milano: Kugler and Ghedini Publ
21. Wullstein S: The epitympanum and ossicular chain. In: Proc International Conference on the Postoperative Evaluation in the Middle Ear Surgery, 14–16 June, Antwerp, 1984. Boston, Dordrecht, Lancaster: Martinus Nijhoff Publ
22. Marquet J: The antro-tympanic interface. In: Proc International Conference on Acute and Secretory Otitis Media, Jerusalem 17–22 November 1985, pp 349–352. Amsterdam: Kugler Publ 1986
23. Lim D, Shimada T, Yoder M: Distribution of mucus secreting cells in normal middle ear mucosa. Arch Otolaryngol 98: 2–9, 1973
24. Aimi K: Role of the tympanic ring in the pathogenesis of congenital cholesteatoma. Laryngoscope 93: 1140–1146, 1983
25. Sadé J, Hadas E: Prognosis evaluation of secretory otitis media as a function of mastoid pneumatization. Arch Otolaryngol 225: 39–44, 1979

MORPHOGENETIC DEVELOPMENT OF MIDDLE EAR FUNCTION IN THE HUMAN FETUS

FRANK F.J. DECLAU*

Department of Otorhinolaryngology (Head: Prof Dr. J. Marquet), University of Antwerp, Wilrijk, Belgium

Introduction

The development of behavioral responses to sound in man appears to occur as early as the 20th fetal week *in utero*[1]. Electrophysiological studies have also noted cortical responses in infants less than 28 weeks gestational age[2]. Consequently, the ability of fetal hearing has aroused our interest in the histiogenesis of the middle ear in relation to its physical properties as an acoustic transformer.

Comprehensive studies have been made on the early embryological development of the middle ear[3-5], on the ossification pattern of the auditory ossicles[6] and also on the aeration of the middle ear cleft[7]. These developmental aspects do not explain completely the establishment of fetal hearing. According to Marquet *et al.*[8] two other concepts are also of main importance for middle ear function and auditory perception: (1) the presence of articulations between the auditory ossicles ensures compensation to sudden static pressure changes or mechanical forces by its visco-elastic properties; (2) the conical form of the tympanic membrane and its attachment to the manubrium mallei are considered as a lever mechanism causing the action of a step-up transformer: this 'membrane transformer' is considered the most important determinant of the impedance matching function of the middle ear, having a greater effect than either the effective ossicular lever ratio or the effective area ratio[9]. Therefore, in order to elucidate morphological maturation of the auditory system, we focus on the following developmental issues: the morphogenetic differentiation of the tympano-ossicular articulations and their ligaments and the formation of a curved tympanic membrane. The latter is closely related to the growth characteristics of the middle ear cleft and this issue will also be investigated in more detail.

Material and methods

The temporal bones of 11 human fetuses were obtained for investigation (Table 1). Fetal age was established by correlating maternal history, crown-rump length, biparietal diameter and head circumference. None of the fetuses involved in this study showed congenital abnormalities. They were preserved by immersion in either unbuffered (pH 5.6−6.2) or phosphate buffered formaldehyde 4% and stored until investigation in the same type of solution at 4°C. The fetal heads were embedded in poly-methyl-methacrylate** and sectioned axially or coronally (parallel or perpen-

* *Correspondence and reprint requests to*: Dr. F. Declau, M.D., ENT Research Laboratory, University of Antwerp, Universiteitsplein 1, B-2610 Wilrijk, Belgium.
** Technovit 3040; Kulzer & Co GmbH, Wehrheim, West-Germany

Middle Ear Structure, Organogenesis and Congenital Defects, pp. 27−39
edited by B. Ars and P. van Cauwenberge
©*1991 Kugler Publications, Amsterdam, New York*

TABLE 1. Age and numbers of specimens studied

No.	Estimated gestational age (weeks)	Sectioning plane of temporal bones
1	14	both coronal
2	16	both coronal
3	18	axial + coronal
4	20	both coronal
5	20	axial + coronal
6	20	both coronal
7	21	axial + coronal
8	22	both coronal
9	23	both coronal
10	25	axial + coronal
11	27	both coronal

dicular to OMBL) through both temporal bones by a semi-automatic cutting system*
so that tissue slices were 1.3 mm thick (tissue loss due to cutting was approximately
400 μm). The 1.3 mm semithin sections obtained could then be worked up for histology by selecting the regions of interest under the operation microscope. When decalcified sections were required, decalcification was performed with either EDTA 0.1 M
(pH 7.4) or 5% trichloroacetic acid. Afterwards, tissue slices were dehydrated and
embedded in paraplast for decalcified sections and in methylmethacrylate (MMA)**
for undecalcified sections. The initial 1.3 mm semi-thin slices were cut on a Leitz or
Jung microtome so that their final thickness was 6 to 8 μm. Staining was performed
by various standard procedures: both undecalcified and decalcified sections were
stained with hematoxylin-phloxin-safranine, trichrome Masson, periodic acid Schiff
and a modified Luxol dye technique as described by Declau et al.[10]. Verhoeff's iron
hematoxylin method was used as a specific stain for elastic tissue. According to the
elegant immunofluorescence study of Pieraggi et al.[11], Verhoeff's stain was most
specific for all components of elastic tissue: elastic, elaunic and oxytalan fibers. In
contrast, orcein stain which has been employed in previous investigations[12,13] gave
an irregular staining reaction with oxytalan fibers.

Observations

Most anatomical and physiological textbooks dismiss the ligaments and the articulations between the auditory ossicles with very brief and incomplete descriptions. To
our knowledge, fetal differentiation of the articulations and of elastic tissue in the
tympano-ossicular system have not been described previously. Davies[12] summarized
the historical descriptions of the elastic tissue component in adult middle ear joints
and gave a very accurate account on its position in those articulations and in the tendons of the stapedius and tensor tympani muscle. Recently, Hartwein and Rauchfuss[14] described the fetal fibrillogenesis of some of the ligaments of the auditory

* Exakt; Walter Messner, Oststeinbeck, West-Germany
** K-Plast; Medim GmbH, Darmstadt, West-Germany

ossicles, but the differentiation of the elastic tissue component has not been investigated.

1. Maturation of articulations, tendons and ligaments

1.1. Synovial articulations

At 14 weeks gestation, the auditory ossicles are entirely cartilaginous, but segmentation has already occurred. The incudo-mallear and incudo-stapedial joints can be identified by their interzone: the interzone is the blastemal condensation that gives rise to the joint cavity and articular ends of the bone. It is visible as a denser stained area between the primitive anlagen of the auditory ossicles. At first the cells of the interzone are identical to those of undifferentiated mesenchyme and differ from the chondrogenic matrix in that they do not form matrix. The fibrous joint capsule originates from the condensed layer of mesenchyme surrounding the future joint, also called synovial mesenchyme; at this stage, the synovial mesenchyme is already vascularized and fibrillogenesis of elastine can be recognized in its inferior part of the primitive incudo-mallear joint. At 16 weeks, not only the incudo-mallear joint, but also the incudo-stapedial joint contain elastic fibers in their synovial mesenchyme. The incudo-stapedial joint seems to contain more elastic fibers superiorly than inferiorly. The elastic fibers pass at right angles to the joint line from the juxta-articular margin of one ossicle to that of the other. At the joint margins the individual elastic fibers diverge to attain a very strong attachment to perichondrium and underlying cartilage. As ossification starts (in malleus and incus: 16 to 17 weeks; stapes: 18 weeks), differentiation of the interzone into three distinct zones becomes visible: a central layer of darker staining cells lies between two zones in which the mesenchymal cells are aligned parallel to the surface of the subjacent cartilage. Cavitation of the joints occurs in the central layer almost immediately thereafter: the amorphous intercellular substance and tissue fluid gradually increase; the cells become widely separated from one another giving rise to multiple spaces which fuse quickly to form the synovial cavity. At the same period, the first synovial lining cells can also be distinguished as flat cells overlying the differentiating synovial mesenchyme. Cavitation occurs centrofugally in the incudo-mallear joint and centropetally in the incudo-stapedial joint. This aspect of joint formation is finished around 23 weeks gestation. The zones adjacent to the cartilage form bundles of collagen in a network fashion parallel to the articular surface and resemble the perichondrium, with which they are continuous; they give both rise to the hyaline articular cartilage. At 23 weeks gestation, three layers can be determined. The superficial layer is composed of small, flat cells parallel to the articular surface. The intermediate layer is made up of the more oval shaped cells and the deep layer consists of large oval or round cells which penetrate into the irregular bone surface.

1.2. Fibrous articulations

1.2.1. Stapedo-vestibular joint. This articulation forms a special type of fibrous articulation: the opposed surfaced of stapes and fenestra vestibuli are connected by fibrocartilage of the elastic variety. At 14 weeks gestational age, the annular ligament

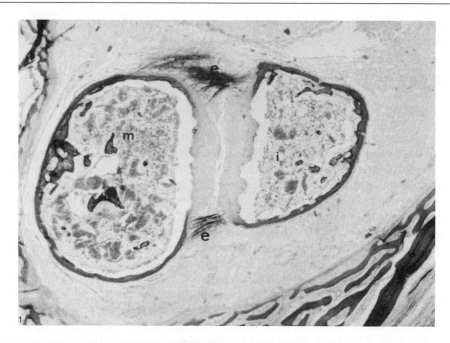

Fig. 1. Joint formation at the incudo (i)-mallear (m) joint at 25 weeks (fetus No. 10; Verhoeff's stain; axial section). Note elastin fibers (e) at the joint capsule. (orig. magn. × 40).

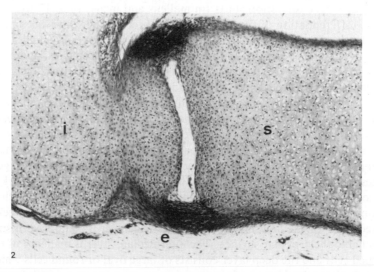

Fig. 2. Joint formation at the incudo (i)-stapedial (s) joint at 20 weeks (fetus No. 6; Verhoeff's stain; coronal section). Note elastin fibers (e) at the joint capsule. (orig. magn. × 33).

consists of undifferentiated mesenchyme without any elastic fibers. The mesenchymal cells have no specific orientation. At 18 weeks, by the time that stapes and vestibular region of the otic capsule become ossified, elastic tissue fibers can be detected. These elastic fibers run parallel to each other and are especially concentrated

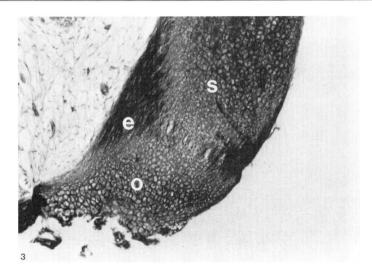

Fig. 3. Joint formation at stapedial (s)-vestibular (o) joint (fetus No. 8; Verhoeff's stain; coronal section). Note elastic fibrocartilage (e). (orig. magn. × 33).

on both sides of the vestibular window where they mix up with the perichondrial membrane. The elastic fibers on the tympanic aspect end within a short distance of the joint; on the contrary, they continue for quite some distance from the joint at the vestibular aspect, particularly posteriorly and they form a compact elastic membrane, lining the cartilage of the stapedial base. The elastic fibers attain firm attachment in the cartilaginous matrix of stapes and vestibular window. At 23 weeks, this fibrocartilaginous articulation contains radially arranged elastic fibers running through a hyaline acellular matrix and penetrating the cartilage on the rim of the base of the stapes and that of the fenestra vestibuli.

1.2.2. Attachment of the anterior malleal process. The anterior malleal process is formed by the goniale, an intra-membranously ossified bone spicule, first detected at 11 weeks[15]. The goniale fuses medially with the malleus around 19 weeks gestational age. At the same period, degeneration of Meckel's cartilage occurs giving rise to the anterior malleal ligament which fixes firmly the anterior malleal process to the petro-tympanic suture. Before its degeneration, Meckel's cartilage is in continuity with the cartilaginous precursor of the malleus. Histologically the cartilaginous ground substance is dissolved centripetally and the cartilaginous cells become fibroblasts producing collagen fibers. No elastic fibers could be detected in this region.

1.2.3. Attachment of the malleus to the tympanic membrane. In contrast to the findings of Harty[13] in adult specimens of the temporal bone, no elastic fibers could be detected in the tympanic membrane nor in its attachment with the manubrium mallei at the fetal period investigated. The manubrium mallei ossifies more slowly than the other parts of the malleus and characteristically hyaline cartilage remains at the lateral malleal process and at the umbo. Even in the 14-week specimen, the attachment of the malleus to the mesenchymatous middle layer of the tympanic membrane consists of condensed mesenchyme. At 18 weeks, the perichondrial membrane

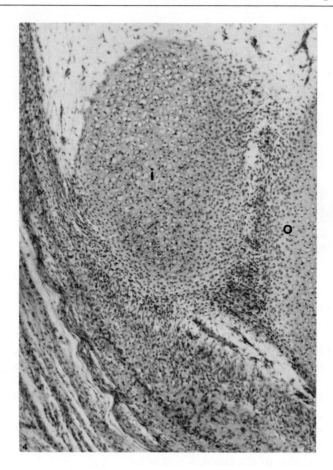

Fig. 4. Pseudo-articulation of the short incudal process (i) with the otic capsule (o) at 14 weeks (fetus No. 1; Verhoeff's stain; coronal section). Ligaments are at the mesenchymal stage. Note mesenchymal condensations at medio-inferior, medio-superior and lateral aspects of the incus. At the lateral portion, mesenchymal tissue is parallel to the cartilaginous process of the incus. In contrast, the medial condensations are already oriented in their final direction. (orig. magn. × 160).

around the manubrium mallei is in continuity with the collagen fibers in the middle layer of the tympanic membrane.

1.2.4. Attachment of the short process of the incus. The medial component of the posterior incudal ligaments attaches the posterior aspect of the incus to the lateral wall of the otic capsule. At 14 weeks, undifferentiated mesenchymal tissue is visible between the cartilaginous matrix of both incus and otic capsule and no elastic fibers can be detected. In the 16-week old fetal specimen, elastic fibers can abundantly be recognized in two regions: (1) between the infero-medial aspect of the incus and a cartilaginous process of the otic capsule: here are most of the elastin fibers situated and (2) between the supero-medial aspect of the incus and the otic capsule also some elastic fibers are found. In between these regions, the cartilaginous matrix of incus and otic capsule are separated by a layer of undifferentiated mesenchymal cells. At

18 weeks, cavitation starts centripetally in this region and the short process of the incus as well as the otic capsule remain cartilaginous in this particular area. At 23 weeks gestation, a mature pseudo-articulation has been formed between the short process of the incus and the lateral wall of the otic capsule surrounded by elastic tissue situated in the so-called medial component of the posterior incudal ligament.

1.3. Tendons of the stapedius and tensor tympani muscle

At 14 gestational weeks, the tendons of both stapedius and tensor tympani muscle already contain collagen fibers. Elastic fibers were first observed at 18.5 weeks in the tendon of the tensor tympani muscle and at 20 weeks in the stapedius tendon. In the M. tensor tympani, elastic fibers were randomly mingled with the collagen fibers of the tendon. In the M. stapedius, elastic tissue was mainly found around the central core of the tendon and within the condensed mesenchyme which is the precursor of the periosteal layer of the pyramid.

1.4. Ligaments

The lateral component of the posterior incudal ligaments can be detected as a condensation of mesenchyme between the supero-lateral aspect of the short process of the incus and pars squamosa at the fossa incudis. The undifferentiated mesenchymal cells run at 14 weeks gestation parallel to the surface of the incus. However, as fibrillogenesis starts at 23 weeks with the formation of collagen and a few scattered elastic fibers, they are oriented in the same way as in the adult ligament.

The superior incudo-malleal ligament[16] is already visible in the 14-week stage as a streak of condensed mesenchyme extending medially from the incudo-mallear capsule to the petro-squamosal suture of the tegmen tympani. Elastic fibers can be detected from 23 weeks gestational age, especially in the region close to the elastic capsule of the incudo-mallear joint. These elastic fibers are mixed with collagen fibers and small blood vessels.

The lateral as well as the posterior malleal ligament are also visible in the 14th-week specimen as a line of condensed mesenchyme between the malleus and pars squamosa in the 14-week-old fetal specimen. Definitive fibrillogenesis is also visible at 23 weeks gestation. Only collagen fibers could be found in these ligaments.

1.5. Secondary tympanic membrane

From 20 weeks gestational age, the future intermediate layer of the secondary tympanic membrane contains abundant elastic fibers. The central portion of this intermediate layer is composed exclusively of elastic fibers while the peripheral margin of the foramen rotundum also contains collagen fibers.

2. Formation of a curved tympanic membrane

The formation of a curved tympanic membrane is inherently attached to the growth movement of the middle ear cleft and of the tympano-ossicular system therein; therefore, it seems reasonable to consider at first middle ear cleft expansion itself.

TABLE 2. Inclination of the tympanic ring (TR) in relation to the ipsilateral semicircular canal (CSL)

Specimen No.	TR ˆCSL left	TR ˆCSL right
1	35°	32°
2	40°	38°
4	36°	37°
8	30°	28°
11	33°	34°

Only a few original papers dealing with the specific growth pattern of the middle ear have been published in the past[7,16,17]. The orientation of the tympanic ring during subsequent developmental stages has also been the subject of a long-standing controversy. Gegenbauer[16] described a gradual verticalization of the tympanic membrane attaining 30 to 35° with reference to the horizontal plane in neonates.

2.1. Growth of the middle ear cleft

2.1.1. Inclination of the tympanic ring. In the present investigation, the orientation of the tympanic ring was not determined in relation to the horizontal plane, but with reference to the ipsilateral otic capsule. Therefore, the angle between the tympanic ring and the plane of the ipsilateral external semicircular canal in coronal macrosections of five fetuses was measured. The same investigation was carried out in an adult control group. On nine coronal CT examinations of normal adult temporal bones, the angulation of the tympanic ring was measured in the same way. The mean value and standard deviation were calculated for both groups: it was respectively 34.3° ± 3.7° for the fetal group and 33.9° ± 3.6° for the adult group (Table 2). In contrast to the gradual verticalization of the tympanic ring in respect to the horizontal plane, its angular relationship to the ipsilateral otic capsule remains essentially the same in both fetal and adult temporal bones.

2.1.2. Growth characteristics of the developing middle ear. The walls of the middle ear cleft are mainly composed of three bony structures: tympanic ring, otic capsule and squamous bone. In early life these primordial parts are not solidly bound by synostoses, but are separated by fibrous planes; this ensures the possibility for their growth and displacement during middle ear cleft expansion. A semi-quantitative analysis of the widening of the middle ear cleft was performed on histological slices of three temporal bones of 14, 20 and 25 weeks (Nos. 1, 4, 10) respectively by means of graphic plotting of the superimposed growth stages. The middle ear cleft was schematized by means of four precisely indicated points forming a quadrangle: (a) the tympanic ring in its inferior part, (b) the inferior end of the pars tympanica ossis squamosi, (c) the petro-squamosal suture and (d) the medial margin of the processus perioticus of the tegmen tympani. A comparative evaluation of the middle ear clefts of these three specimens reveals a gradual enlargement with a factor 1.67 between the 14th and 20th and of 1.56 between the 20th and 25th week. Expansion of the middle ear cleft consists of two basically different modes: (1) intrinsic growth and remodelling of its constituents and (2) lateral displacement of the squamous bone and tympanic ring with respect to the otic capsule. The intrinsic growth is most clearly

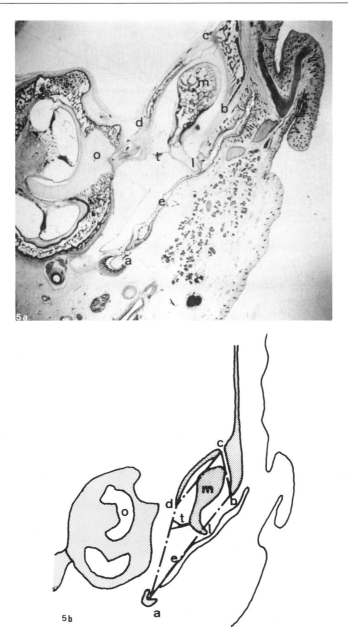

Fig. 5a,b. Topography of the middle ear cleft in a 20-week fetus (No. 4; coronal section, left side; Verhoeff's stain). o : otic capsule; a : tympanic ring; b : inferior end of pars tympanica ossis squamosi; c : petro-squamosal suture; d : medial end of processus perioticus tegminis tympani; m : malleus; t: M. tensor tympani; l : processus lateralis mallei; e : tympanic membrane.

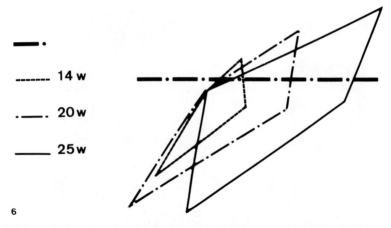

Fig. 6. Schematised representation of the middle ear cleft in three subsequent growth stages: 14, 20 and 25 weeks. •—•: plane of the ipsilateral external semicircular canal.

demonstrated by the enlargement of the diameter of the tympanic ring. Between the 14th and 20th weeks, this diameter increases with 2.6 mm (from 5.0 to 7.6 mm) and between the 20th and 25th weeks with only 0.6 mm (from 7.6 to 8.2 mm); this gradual increase in size is caused by drift — a continuous remodelling process by the characteristic combination of bone resorption at its inner side by osteoclasts and bone deposition at its outer side by osteoblasts. The lateral displacement of the squamous bone is primarily due to the growth pressure of the enlarging brain upon the skull. The squamous bone and the petrosquamosal suture are displaced in a supero-lateral direction of ± 25° with reference to the plane of the ipsilateral external semicircular canal; the displacement between the 14th and 25th week with respect to the otic capsule amounts to 6.2 mm! This growth movement is accompanied by remodelling and growth of the squamous bone. In order to follow the lateral displacement of the latter, the periotic process broadens in a proportional way. The overall growth process leads to an enlargement and altered shape of the epitympanic space. In contrast to the squamous bone, the tympanic ring is displaced laterally, parallel to the plane of the ipsilateral external semicircular canal; its displacement between the 14th and 25th week amounts to 4.1 mm. Drift and lateral displacement act simultaneously on the tympanic ring in divergent directions. Between the 14th and 20th week, one neutralizes the other in such a way that the inferior region of the middle ear cleft keeps its original shape. Between the 20th and 25th week, however, the growth movement by lateral displacement is far more important than drift (2.45 mm versus 0.6 mm respectively); its resultant vector (drift + lateral displacement) is directed inferolaterally with respect to the ipsilateral external semicircular canal (−10°). Consequently, the tympanic ring separates from the otic capsule and leads to the formation of the hypotympanum.

2.2. Growth characteristics of the tympano-ossicular system

Throughout the fetal period studied, the characteristic shape of the malleus is preserved; its length increases by a factor 1.75 between 14 and 20 weeks gestational age, but remains unchanged at the 20th and 25th week. The increase in size is due

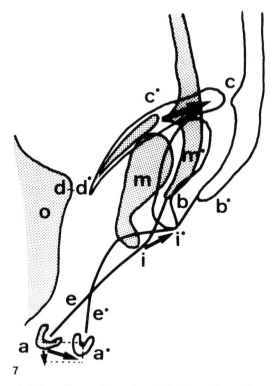

Fig. 7. Growth movement of the malleus and curvature of the tympanic membrane. Superimposed draw-
ing of a coronal section of the middle ear at 20 (No. 4) and 25 weeks (No. 10). Shaded area at 20 weeks.

to the intrinsic growth and remodelling of the cartilaginous matrix. At 16 weeks,
when the cartilaginous precursor has reached 'adult' proportions, ossification starts
in the malleus neck by endochondral bone formation. The entire malleus undergoes
lateral displacement with the same direction as the petro-squamosal suture. This is
not surprising since the superior incudo-malleal ligament connects the incudo-
mallear joint capsule with this suture. Since the malleus is intimately connected with
the tympanic membrane, the growth movement of the processus lateralis of the
malleus was studied with particular attention. Between 14 and 20 weeks, its ultimate
displacement is the resultant of two diverging growth vectors: (1) the intrinsic growth
of the cartilaginous matrix which starts ossification in the 16th-week specimen and
(2) lateral displacement, in a direction similar to that of the petro-squamosal suture
but one half of its magnitude; the resultant vector is almost identical to the lateral
displacement of the tympanic membrane. The position of the processus lateralis
mallei within the tympanic membrane has been established by the distance ratio
b$-1/1-$a; this ratio remains identical in both specimens (0.40 at 14 weeks and 0.47
at 20 weeks) and the tympanic membrane keeps a planar shape.

   Between the 20th and 25th week of intrauterine life, when the malleus has reached
adult proportions, its growth movement is solely due to lateral displacement in a
supero-lateral direction of 25°, identical to the petro-squamosal suture. Since the
growth vectors of the tympanic membrane ($-10°$) and of the malleus ($+25°$) diverge,

the processus lateralis of the malleus is relocated within the tympanic membrane (b − 1/1 − a : 0.19 at 25 weeks). The tympanic membrane gradually develops a cone-shaped aspect because it displaces relatively more than the malleus handle to which it is intimately related.

Discussion

Our results present a developing system in which each developmental stage merges into the others, influences subsequent stages and must occur in the proper sequence and in proper temporal relationship with other aspects of development; only by these developmental characteristics does the auditory system become progressively more competent at responding to the full range of sound stimuli.

Interpretation of these complex developmental aspects results in a better under-standing of basic physiological mechanisms of adult middle ear function. In contrast to the development of other joints in the human fetus, the differentiation of articulations between the auditory ossicles starts only in the fetal period. Maturation of the articulations is attained around 23 weeks gestational age. Another peculiarity is the presence of an 'incudo-labyrinthic joint' between the short process of the incus and the otic capsule, containing abundant elastic fibers. Abundant elastic fibers are also present within the joint capsule of the incudo-mallear, incudo-stapedial articulations and in the fibrocartilage of the stapedo-vestibular joint. The dynamic elastic properties of the elastin molecule seem very peculiar[18] in view of its presence in the articulations of the auditory ossicles: its resilience drops off very rapidly at frequencies above about 10 Hz. This drop in resilience is the indication of a shift in properties, called the glass transition. This means that when acoustic energy enters the middle ear (frequencies > 10 Hz), the elastin behaves as a rigid tissue and the ossicular system will act as one unit. In cases of static pressure differences (with frequencies < 10 Hz) however, the elastin will behave as an elastic tissue and protect the inner ear by changing the configuration of the tympano-ossicular system.

From our morphological observations, gradual maturation of the membrane transformer is established around 25 weeks gestational age. Its maturation is the result of growth cleft enlargement and the growth movement of the malleus therein. Around the same period, aeration of the mesotympanum is almost completed and the meatal plug, forming the primitive external ear canal, has gradually opened[19]. Consequently, at this fetal period maturation of the middle ear has reached almost completion and its physiological ability becomes possible not only as an impedance matching system but also as a protective device for inner ear function.

References

1. Ruben R, Rapin I: Plasticity of the developing auditory system. Ann Otol 89: 303–311, 1980
2. Graziani LJ, Weitzman ED, Velasco MSA: Neurologic maturation and auditory evoked responses in low birth weight infants. Pediatrics 41: 483–494, 1968
3. Hanson JR, Anson BJ, Strickland EM: Branchial sources of the auditory ossicles in Man: observations of embryonic stages from 7 mm to 28 mm. Arch Otolaryngol 76: 200–215, 1962
4. Eyries C, Perles B: Embryologie de l'oreille. In: *Encyclopédie Médico-chirurgicale d'Otorhinolaryngologie*, 20005: A10–A30. Paris 1980

5. Van de Water TR, Maderson PFA, Jaskoll TF: The morphogenesis of the middle and external ear. Birth Def 16(4): 147–180, 1980
6. Anson BJ, Bast TH, Cauldwell EW: The development of the auditory ossicles, the otic capsule and extracapsular tissue. Ann Otol Rhinol Laryngol 60: 957–985, 1947
7. Proctor B: Chronic otitis media and mastoiditis. In: *Otolaryngology*, Vol 2. Paparella M, Shumrick D (eds). Philadelphia: WB Saunders 1980
8. Marquet J, Van Camp KJ, Creten WL, Decraemer WF, Wolff HB: Topics in physics and middle ear surgery. Acta Oto-Rhino-Laryngol Belg 27: 137–320, 1973
9. Tonndorf J, Khanna SM: The role of the tympanic membrane in middle ear transmission. Ann Otolaryngol 79: 743, 1970
10. Declau F, Moeneclaey L, Marquet J: A new indication for Luxol fast blue stain: differentiation of cartilage and bone in human fetal temporal bones. Arch Oto-Rhino-Laryngol 245: 218–220, 1988
11. Pieraggi MT, Nejjar I, Julian M, Bouissou H: Staining of elastic tissue by Verhoeff's iron hematoxylin. Ann Pathol 6(1): 74–77, 1986
12. Davies DV: A note on the articulations of the auditory ossicles and related structures. J Laryngol Otol 62: 533–536, 1948
13. Harty M: Elastic tissue in the middle ear cavity. J Laryngol Otol 67: 723–729, 1953
14. Hartwein JHJ, Rauchfuss A: The development of the ossicular ligaments in the human middle ear. Arch Oto-Rhino-Laryngol 244: 23–25, 1987
15. Marquet J: The incudo-malleal joint. J Laryngol Otol 95: 543–565, 1981
16. Gegenbauer C (ed): *Traité d'Anatomie humain*. Leipzig: Von Wilhelm Engelman 1883
17. Bok HE: *De Foetale Transformatie van het Middenoorgebied*. Amsterdam: Drukkerij Holland 1966
18. Gosline JM, Rosenbloom J: Elastin. In: *Extracellular Matrix Biochemistry*. Piez KA, Reddy AM (eds). New York: Elsevier 1984
19. Michaels L: Development of the stratified squamous epithelium of the human tympanic membrane and external canal: the origin of auditory epithelial migration. Am J Anat 184: 334–344, 1989

DEVELOPMENTAL ASPECTS OF THE FACIAL CANAL

FRANK F.J. DECLAU*

Department of Otorhinolaryngology (Head: Prof Dr J Marquet), University of Antwerp, Wilrijk, Belgium

Introduction

Otologic surgeons require more detailed information on the relationship of the facial nerve to its bony canal and on developmental events whose disruption can result in anomalies of the facial nerve (Fallopian) canal[1].

Most anatomical and embryological textbooks dismiss the development of the facial canal with very brief and incomplete descriptions. Whereas dehiscences have been attributed to persistence of the stapedial artery[2] or middle ear infections in early childhood[3], most authors believe that the normal formation of a closed facial canal is entirely the result of otic capsule ossification. However, post-mortem temporal bone studies of Marquet[4] have demonstrated preferential sites for facial canal dehiscences. Most frequently dehiscences were found in the vestibular region of the tympanic segment (12%). In contrast, dehiscences were very rare in the cochlear region of the tympanic segment (only 1%). In the labyrinthine segment, a prevalence of 7% was found. These observations suggest a more complex way of facial canal development which cannot be entirely explained by otic capsule ossification.

Material and methods

In order to explain the preferential sites of facial dehiscences, the ossification pattern of the otic capsule was investigated in fetal temporal bones with both light and scanning electron microscopy. Fetal age was correlated to maternal history, crown-rump length, biparietal diameter and head circumference. None of the fetuses showed congenital abnormalities. Twenty-two temporal bones were studied by means of light microscopy. The fetal heads were preserved in 4% buffered formaldehyde. They were then embedded in poly-methyl-methacrylate** and sectioned coronally or axially through both temporal bones by a semi-automatic cutting system◇ so that tissue slices were 1.3 mm thick. Afterwards, sections were decalcified with 5% trichloroacetic acid or 0.1 M EDTA, dehydrated and embedded in paraplast or methyl-methacrylate◇◇. The initial 1.3 mm semithin sections were cut on a Leitz microtome so that their final thickness was 8 μm. They were stained by means of various staining procedures: hematoxylin-phloxin-safranine stain, trichome Masson stain, periodic acid Schiff reaction, Sirius red F3BA stain and a modified Luxol dye technique, described previously by Declau et al.[5].

* *Correspondence and reprint requests to*: Dr F Declau, M.D., ENT Research Laboratory, University of Antwerp, Universiteitsplein 1, B-2610 Wilrijk, Belgium
** Technovit 714; Kulzer & Co GmbH, Wehrheim, FRG
◇ Exakt; Walter Messner, Oberflächentechnik, Barsbütteler Weg 6, Oststeinbeck, FRG
◇◇ K-plast; Medim GmbH, Darmstadt, FRG

Middle Ear Structure, Organogenesis and Congenital Defects, pp. 41–48
edited by B. Ars and P. van Cauwenberge
©*1991 Kugler Publications, Amsterdam, New York*

TABLE 1. Age and numbers of specimens studied

No.	Estimated gestational age (weeks)	Sectioning plane of temporal bones	Type of investigation
1	14	both coronal	LM
2	16	both coronal	LM
3	18	axial + coronal	LM
4	20	both coronal	LM
5	20	axial + coronal	LM
6	20	both coronal	LM
7	21	axial + coronal	LM
8	21	–	SEM
9	22	both coronal	LM
10	22	–	SEM
11	23	both coronal	LM
12	25	axial + coronal	LM
13	25	both coronal	LM

In order to reveal the fine structure of bone, additionally four complete fetal temporal bones were treated with sodium hypochlorite according to the method described by Boyde et al.[6]. These inorganic specimens were coated with carbon and investigated with a scanning electron microscope (Jeol 733 superprobe, 10KeV, 1nA).

Observations

In order to reveal the effect of otic capsule ossification on facial canal development, all observations were carried out on fetuses between 14 and 25 weeks gestational age. Not only the histological features of the facial canal will be described, but also its topographical characteristics. These observations permitted us to distinguish three phases in facial canal development during the critical period of otic capsule ossification.

1. Phase 1: until 16 weeks gestational age

1.1. Histological considerations. Until 16 weeks gestation, the otic capsule is still completely cartilaginous. Along its entire intratemporal course, the perichondrium of the primitive cartilaginous otic capsule splits around the facial nerve. The perichondrium forms a sort of connective tissue-like frame of condensed mesenchyme around the neural fiber bundle. This 'frame' contains spindle-shaped undifferentiated cells and is clearly different from the epineural sheet.

1.2. Fetal anatomy. In its intrameatal portion, the facial nerve is in close relation with the superior branch of the vestibular nerve and is completely surrounded by primitive cartilaginous matrix. The facial nerve then enters the labyrinthine segment which is situated between the cochlear apex anteriorly and vestibular space posteriorly. This segment of the facial canal consists of a narrow slit situated within the primitive cartilage of the otic capsule: the facial canal is completely dehiscent towards the

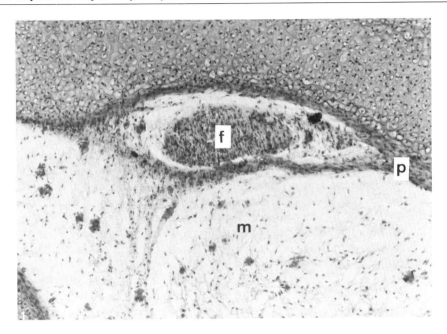

Fig. 1. Facial canal at the vestibular portion of the tympanic segment at 14 weeks gestation. HFS-stain, orig. magn. × 160, fetus No. 1. The facial canal is merely a shallow sulcus at the tympanic side of the cartilaginous otic capsule. The facial nerve (f) is not covered by bone and is in close relation to the mesenchyme of the middle ear cleft (m). The perichondrium of the otic capsule (p) splits around the facial nerve as a connective tissue-like frame.

middle cranial fossa and is covered only by condensed mesenchymal tissue. This area includes the geniculate ganglion, also characterized by direct dural attachment to its epineurium. At the geniculate ganglion area, the facial nerve makes a sharp right-angled turn backward to enter the tympanic segment. The cochlear portion of the tympanic segment is also partially situated within the fossa media and completely dehiscent towards the brain. The facial nerve courses peripherally from the middle cranial fossa to the middle ear through an opening in the pars membranacea tegminis tympani, also known as the primitive hiatus of the facial canal. This fibrous slit is formed by the otic capsule medially and the periotic process laterally. The roof of the middle ear cleft has indeed a complex origin, from lateral to medial we observe: (a) pars tegmentalis squamosi: a bony part of the os squamosum, (b) processus perioticus: an antero-frontal cartilaginous process from the canalicular pool of the otic capsule and (c) pars membranacea tegminis tympani which forms a fibrous hiatus between the periotic process and the otic capsule. The nerve proceeds in the middle ear as the vestibular portion of the tympanic segment and lies in a shallow groove which is totally dehiscent towards the middle ear cleft. The facial sulcus increases progressively in size due to the intrinsic growth and remodelling of the cartilaginous matrix. In the region of the stapedial muscle, the facial sulcus widens, giving space for the anlagen of the facial recess laterally and the sinus tympani medially. The facial nerve and stapedial muscle are also separated from the surrounding mesenchyme by a collagen producing layer. At the base of the stapedial muscle, a

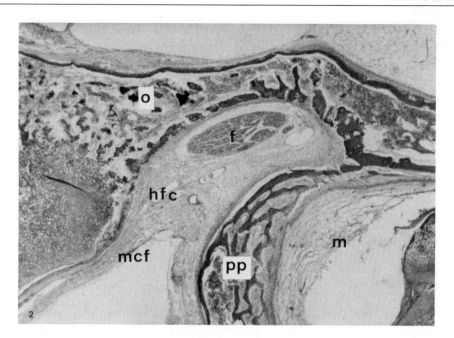

Fig. 2. Hiatus of the facial canal at 18 weeks gestation. HFS-stain, orig. magn. × 62, fetus No. 3. The facial nerve (f) passes through an opening of the pars membranacea tegminis tympani (hfc) from the middle cranial fossa (mcf) into the middle ear cleft (m). The facial nerve is surrounded by endochondral bone of the otic capsule (o) and the periotic process (pp).

cartilaginous bar, Reichert's cartilage, is evident: it participates here in the formation of a portion of the Fallopian canal wall. This second arch cartilage runs first from the lateral side of the otic capsule medially and then in a fronto-caudal direction. The facial nerve runs from behind to the lateral side of Reichert's cartilage into the retromandibular region.

2. Phase 2: 16–21 weeks gestational age

2.1. Histological considerations. In the 16-week specimen, ossification of the otic capsule has started at different ossification centers. The otic capsule ossifies by replacement of the cartilage by endochondral bone. At its inner and outer side, this type of bone is covered by an inner and outer layer of periosteal bone. Wherever the facial nerve is in contact with the otic capsule, periosteal bone formation is lacking initially. The deep sheet of the perichondrial membrane differentiates into a periosteum but bone formation is delayed. Fibrillogenesis has increased to produce a distinct semi-circle. This periosteum consists of two layers: a cellular one in close contact with the endochondral layer containing undifferentiated cells and a fibrous one containing collagen fibers. At the outer sheet, no signs of ossification can be found. There are abundant collagen fibers due to advanced fibrillogenesis of collagen and a few undifferentiated cells can be observed.

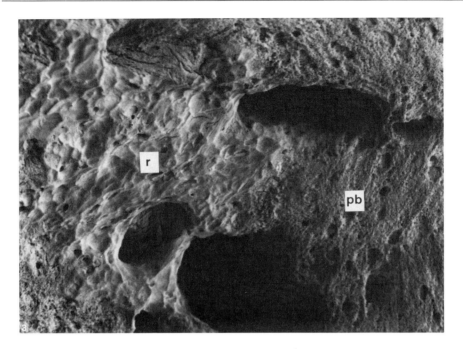

Fig. 3. SEM picture of the inner side of the facial canal in the vestibular portion of the tympanic segment at 22 weeks (orig. magn. × 600, fetus No. 10). In continuity with the periosteal bone (pb) of the fetal woven type, resorption bays (r) can be noted. A combined process of bone secretion and resorption seems responsible for the final architecture of the facial canal.

2.2. Fetal anatomy. The labyrinthine segment is still completely dehiscent towards the middle fossa. At the primitive hiatus of the facial canal, the cartilaginous matrix of the otic capsule and periotic process is now ossified in endochondral bone. The primitive cartilage around the facial sulcus of the tympanic segment is also transformed into endochondral bone. At the second bend of the facial canal where the facial nerve is accompanied by the stapedius muscle, the otic capsule is cartilaginous and the facial canal has the same histological properties as in the phase 1 era. This region of the facial canal is the last to ossify.

3. Phase 3: 22–25 weeks gestational age

3.1. Histological considerations. The facial canal comes to lie deeper in the otic capsule due to the surrounding periosteal bone investment. Details of the closing facial canal demonstrate intra-membranous ossification at its tympanic border: osteoid is secreted by differentiating osteoblasts forming primitive bone of the coarse bundle type. This type of ossification process originates from the bony periosteal edges. Between these clasps of the gradually closing facial canal, a so-called aplastic zone is visible. The luminal side of the facial canal acquires a periosteal investment in continuity with the underlying endochondral bone: primitive bone of the woven type is deposited onto the endochondral bone spicules of the otic capsule. This type of bone is characterized by the presence of many irregularly shaped lacunae and an

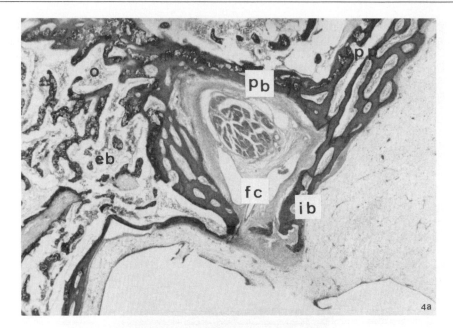

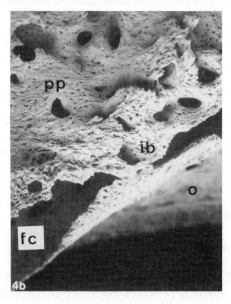

Fig. 4a,b. Facial canal at the cochlear portion of the tympanic segment at phase 3. Fig 4a: HFS-stain, orig. magn. × 62, fetus No. 12; Fig 4b: SEM, orig. magn. × 100, fetus No. 10. The primitive hiatus of the facial canal has been closed. The luminal side of the facial canal (fc) acquires a periosteal bone investment (pb), laid down on the endochondral bone spicules (eb) of the otic capsule (o). At the site of the periotic process (pp), also periosteal bone of the woven type can be observed. The bony clasps closing the facial canal in this region constitute intra-membranous bone (ib) of the coarse bundle type.

at random organization of the collagen matrix. In the region of the second bend of the facial canal, a region of resorption instead of bone formation was found and also a few osteoclasts were observed here. The meaning of this dynamic process is not clear at the moment.

3.2. Fetal anatomy. The labyrinthine segment remains completely dehiscent towards the middle cranial fossa. At the opening in the pars membranacea tegminis tympani where the facial nerve enters the middle ear, the facial canal is closed by bone due to the intramembranous formation of two bony ledges: these bony ledges are situated at the infero-lateral border of the pars membranacea tegminis tympani: they extend from the infero-medial border of the periotic process and at the otic capsule from the infero-lateral border of the facial sulcus. As these bony plates begin to approach each other, they effectively close the primitive hiatus under the facial nerve and separate the epitympanum from the middle cranial fossa. From this area, the facial canal progressively closes posteriorwards to the vestibular region of the tympanic segment by means of intramembranous ossification. In the second bend, formation of the pyramidal process is also initiated as well as the bony wall separating the facial nerve and stapedius muscle.

Discussion

Our observations confirm the physiologic presence of fetal dehiscences. Their locations in fetuses were precisely circumscribed and depend on both their topographic relationship with the otic capsule and its degree of maturation. The intratympanic part of the facial canal and the geniculate ganglion area were the last regions to be covered by bone. The formation of a facial canal is more complex than is generally believed. The complex development of the facial canal is not limited to the 'simple' ossification of the otic capsule as previously described by other authors[7,8]. Endochondral ossification of the otic capsule does not virtually change the shape of the primitive facial sulcus found in the previous cartilage stages: the facial nerve remains widely dehiscent and only covered by a thin fibrous layer. Our observations confirm the importance of the inner and outer connective-tissue sheets around the facial canal: these fibrous layers seem to be responsible for its final architecture and not the otic capsule ossification by itself. Their time sequence is equally important: first, periosteal ossification is delayed at the inner fibrous layer while the side walls acquire a periosteal investment in continuity with the underlying endochondral bone. Consequently, the shape of the facial sulcus is altered. As periosteal ossification is started in the inner sheet, intramembranous bone is formed within the outer fibrous sheet and results in the final closure of the facial canal wall. In the geniculate ganglion area, intramembranous ossification of the fibrous layer situated under the dura mater of the middle cranial fossa is delayed until childhood resulting in dehiscences at this area in 7% of adults[4]: it is called after Von Spee[9] the hiatus of the facial canal.

Kaplan *et al.*[2] have suggested as a possible cause for dehiscences, persistence of the aperture for the stapedial artery which itself disappears at the tenth week. Abing *et al.*[3] have stressed the possibility of middle ear infections in early infancy as a cause for dehiscences. It is evident that neither the persistence of the aperture for the stapedial artery, nor infections in the middle ear explain these observations in widely different topographic regions. Our findings show that those regions of the facial canal wall which are covered by intramembranous bone are the most susceptible to dehiscences, which is totally in agreement with the dehiscence rate found in adults. In time sequence, it is the type of bone which is the last to be formed in order to close the facial canal wall.

Intramembranous ossification constitutes bone formation within connective tissue; this connective tissue contains fibroblasts which are differentiated from neural crest-derived mesenchyme[10]. These crest cells in the head have been shown to undergo osteogenesis in response to close association with embryonic epithelia or their extracellular matrix products. After epigenetic triggering of these mesenchymal cells, a cascade of cellular changes is initiated that ultimately results in the differentiation of osteoblasts, formation of osteoid and deposition of calcium salts[11]. The precise molecular mechanisms underlying these sequences are not known but seem to be highly specific and structured. According to Piez and Reddy[12], a role for both collagens and glycosaminoglycans has been implied.

Disruption of epithelial-mesenchymal tissue interactions can explain the occurrence of dehiscences. The regions which ossify in membranous bone are always in intimate relation with epithelia: *in casu*, middle ear mucosa and arachnoid membrane; disturbances in these tissue relationships may lead to inadequate osteogenesis and may explain why clinically a much higher incidence of dehiscences is found in cases of severe congenital middle ear malformations[13]. In these cases the facial nerve is only covered by a primitive connective tissue layer.

References

1. Ralli G, Ars B, Pafundi E. Natural bony dehiscences in the tympanic segment of the adult fallopian canal. In: Proceedings of the International Symposium of the Politzer Society. Amsterdam: Kugler Publications 1990
2. Kaplan S, Catlin F, Weavert T, Feigin R: Onset of hearing loss in children with bacterial meningitis. Pediatrics 73: 575–578, 1984
3. Abing W, Rauchfuss A: Fetal development of the tympanic part of the facial canal. Arch ORL 243: 374–377, 1987
4. Marquet J: Congenital malformations and middle ear surgery. J Roy Soc Med 74: 119–128, 1981
5. Declau F, Moeneclaey L, Forton G, Marquet J: Differentiation of cartilage and bone in human fetal temporal bones with Luxol fast blue stain. Arch ORL 245: 218–220, 1988
6. Boyde A, Maconnachie E, Reid SA, Delling G, Mundy G: Scanning electron microscopy in bone pathology: review of methods, potential and applications. Scanning Electron Microscopy 4: 1537–1554, 1986
7. Bast T: Ossification of the otic capsule in human fetuses. Carnegie Contr to Embryol 121: 53–82, 1930
8. Broman J: Die Entwicklungsgeschichte der Gehörknöchelchen. Anat Hefte 11: 59–670, 1899
9. Von Spee F (ed): Skeletlehre: *Kopf. Handbuch der Anatomie von Menschen*. Jena: Fisher Verlag 1896
10. Weston A, Ciment G, Girdlestone J: The role of extracellular matrix in neural crest development: a reevaluation. In: *The Role of Extracellular Matrix in Development*. New York: Allan R Liss 1984
11. Hall B: Genetic and epigenetic control of connective tissues in the craniofacial structures. Birth Def 20(3): 1–17, 1984
12. Piez K, Reddy A (eds): *Extracellular Matrix Biochemistry*. New York: Elsevier 1984
13. Marquet J, Declau F (eds): Congenital middle ear malformations. Acta ORL Belg 42(2): 123–302, 1988

STRATIFIED SQUAMOUS EPITHELIUM IN RELATION TO THE TYMPANIC MEMBRANE
Its development and kinetics

LESLIE MICHAELS[1] and SAVA SOUCEK[2]

[1] *Department of Histopathology, University College and Middlesex School of Medicine, Institute of Laryngology and Otology, 330 Gray's Inn Road, London, WC1X 8EE;* [2] *ENT/Audiology Department, St. Mary's Hospital, Praed Street, London, W2 1NY, UK*

Introduction

This paper is concerned with the stratified squamous epithelium of the eardrum which occurs not only as the lining of the outer surface, but also as a developmental rest at the edge of the inner.

The epithelium of the middle ear is a single flat layer while that of the Eustachian tube is columnar and pseudostratified. The cell rest of stratified squamous epithelium, the epidermoid formation (EF), is seen in most fetal ears at the junction of those epithelia, at the anterior edge of the tympanic membrane until 33 weeks gestation, when it disappears[1,2]. Its origin can be traced to early embryonic life when it arises, perhaps, from the ectoderm of the first branchial groove. It is likely that congenital cholesteatoma in the anterior superior position is derived from the EF by its continued growth instead of regression[3,4].

The stratified squamous epithelium on the outer side of the tympanic membrane has an activity which is unique. It moves or migrates laterally. Migration is a physiological function of the epithelium of the tympanic membrane which is necessary to cleanse the membrane from the otherwise inevitable build-up of keratin so as to allow delicate vibration for transmission of sound impulses. The daubing of dye on the tympanic membrane and its subsequent repeated observation is a convenient method for plotting the movement of the stratified squamous epithelium. Pathways of movement studied in this way have been described by several observers. Stinson[5] found that movement was from anterior to posterior. Other observers[6,7] found that dye moved radially from the umbo to the periphery.

The photographs of the dye movement made previously[6,7] were obtained through an ear speculum from the outside. The recent advent of the Hopkins rod lens system has allowed a close-up wide angle photograph of the whole of the eardrum to be taken after advancing the tip of the endoscope past the narrow isthmus of the external canal. This system provides also a closer and therefore a clearer view of both normal landmarks and any dye-markings that may have been daubed on the eardrum. We carried out a study of the pathways of migration on the human tympanic membrane in which we have used serial photographs taken by this modern system to follow the movements of dye-markings[8]. In the present paper we summarize the results of these findings.

We believe that this unidirectional flow of epithelium in auditory epithelial migration must have its origin in the early formation of the stratified squamous epithelium

Middle Ear Structure, Organogenesis and Congenital Defects, pp. 49–55
edited by B. Ars and P. van Cauwenberge
©*1991 Kugler Publications, Amsterdam, New York*

of the tympanic membrane and external canal. We analyzed the structure of this epithelium in the course of embryonic, fetal and postnatal development in both the human and the mouse and have indeed been able to explain the source of auditory epithelial migration as a continuous embryologic growth persisting into maturity. The patterns of the developing epithelia have also contributed to some degree towards an understanding of the mechanism of the migratory activity. An outline of these developmental findings will also be presented.

Materials and methods

Pathways of migration in the living tympanic membrane

To study the normally occurring movement of epithelium on the tympanic membrane, 24 ears of eight female and four male volunteers of ages 21 to 63, all without a history of ear disease, were used. The membranes were daubed with Bonney's Blue, a mixture of 1% crystal violet and 1% brilliant green solutions in 90% alcohol. This mixture is regularly used in dermatological practice in the United Kingdom. The dye was placed on the appropriate part of the eardrum through an ear speculum with a fine cotton-tipped metal ear probe, under magnification of an operating microscope.

Developmental studies in relation to migratory activity

To study the development of the tympanic membrane in the embryonic human ear 12 ears from six embryos were examined in serial sections. Embryos were embedded in paraffin wax after being oriented for cutting either in a horizontal or in a coronal plane and serial sections were cut at $4-6$ μm. A variety of stains was used including hematoxylin and eosin, Masson's trichrome and Bodian's silver stain.

For the fetal and mature human ear histological sections of 167 post-mortem ears from 117 cases ranging from 45 days gestation to adult life were examined. Earlier specimens were of the whole head which was fixed in 10% buffered formaldehyde solution soon after delivery, decalcified, embedded in low viscosity nitrocellulose or paraffin wax and horizontally sectioned at 20 μm. Every tenth section was mounted and stained with hematoxylin and eosin. In older specimens the temporal bone only was cut, embedded in low viscosity nitrocellulose or paraffin wax and horizontally sectioned at 20 μm.

124 ears from 72 mice of mixed, interbred strains and both sexes, at stages of development ranging from embryos at 11 gestational days to mature animals at 100 days were examined. In most of them both ears were examined, the whole head having been serially sectioned in a transverse plane.

Results

Pathways of migration in the living tympanic membrane

There are two pathways of dye movement on the tympanic membrane. In the pars flaccida (PF) region movement is always posterior and superior to the adjacent deep

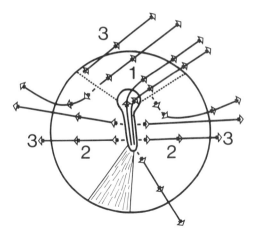

Fig. 1. Diagram to show pathways of movement on the eardrum. Zone 1: over handle of malleus superiorly and then posterosuperiorly over whole pars flaccida to zone 3 (deep external canal). Zone 2: away from pars flaccida and handle of malleus region radially across pars tensa region (zone 2) to zone 3 (deep external canal).

external canal. On the handle of the malleus (HM) surface dye always moves upwards along the line of the handle to the lateral process of the malleus and then posteriorly and superiorly on the PF pathway. The stratified squamous epithelium on the PF and the HM together constitute a separate epithelial area which we have called zone 1 (see below).

Pars tensa (PT) migration shows a different pathway. In front of the lateral process dye moves anteriorly and superiorly; behind the lateral process dye moves posteriorly and superiorly. Approximately in the region of the edge of the HM dye moves anteriorly, posteriorly or inferiorly across the PT in the shortest crossing to the rim of the eardrum. Thus the movement of the PT is quite separate from that of the PF and HM regions and is radial and centrifugal. The stratified squamous epithelium on the PT constitutes another separate epithelial area which we have called zone 2 (see below) (Fig. 1).

Development of stratified squamous epithelium (Fig. 2)

The epithelium of the external auditory canal and tympanic membrane in the human and in the mouse develop along similar lines[8,9]. When the primary external canal (first branchial groove) has been formed (at five weeks in the human and 12 days in the mouse) its fundus is composed of a flatter epithelium than that lining its side walls. The fundal epithelium is a precursor of zone 1, which lines the PF and HM regions and the side walls, that of zone 4, lining the cartilaginous canal. Serial sections reveal the shape of the fundal region to be wide above and narrow below to conform to the primordial head and HM. Two folds arise from the epithelium at the edge of the fundus. One fold, emanating from around a large proportion of the circumference, is the meatal plate (MP) first described by Hammar[10]. It grows in the direction of the tubotympanic recess, eventually to lie alongside it. The epithelium of the MP is precisely structured with regard to thick and thin regions. The medial

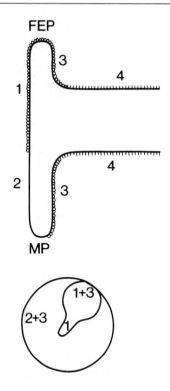

Fig. 2. Diagram of early external canal and eardrum. Above a diagram of a horizontal section can be seen and below a diagram of an *en face* view of the eardrum. 1, 2, 3 and 4: zones of epithelium; FEP: fundal extension plate; MP: meatal plate. For description please see text.

epithelium of the fold comprising the MP becomes very thin and eventually forms the external covering of the PT. We have called this epithelium zone 2. The lateral epithelium of the MP becomes the covering of the adjacent deep external canal (zone 3). The epithelium between zone 2 and 3 is particularly thick (see below).

The second fold is not as prominent in humans as in mice. It grows from the remainder of the edge of the fundus of the primary canal which had not contributed to the MP. We have referred to this fold as the fundal extension plate (FEP). The medial aspect of the FEP with the whole of the fundal epithelium comes to cover the pars flaccida (PF) and the HM and its lateral aspect the adjacent deep canal (zone 3). The epithelium of the side walls of the primary external canal develops into that of the cartilaginous canal (zone 4).

The next stage, which is one of opening up and clearing of the deep canal and meatal plate, commences in the human at 18 weeks gestation and in the mouse at eight days after birth, in both cases at the same time as cornification of the stratified squamous epithelium of the external canal. Zones 2 and 3 are in continuity along the rim of the tympanic membrane.

The final stage involving widening of the whole canal is a process which is prominent in later fetal life and continues until adult life. Flattening of all the epithelia occurs but stratified squamous epithelium in zones 1 and 3 is still thicker than in zone 2, a state of affairs which persists throughout life[9].

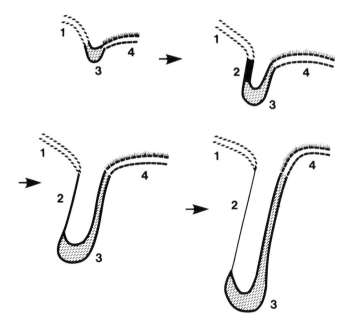

Fig. 3. Early development of mouse meatal plate from 13th gestational day at top left to 17th gestational day at bottom right. For description please see text.

Early development of the meatal plate

The early development of the MP in the mouse has been observed by us in daily sequence. Commencing as an ingrowth of cells with marked mitotic activity at the junction of zone 1 and zone 4 the MP becomes elongated towards the tubotympanic recess. As it does so, the marked thickening and mitotic activity of cells persist at its tip and to a lesser extent on the external side of the MP, representing zone 3, but there is a progressive attenuation of the internal layer of the MP (zone 2), which becomes extremely thin and flattened (Fig. 3).

Discussion

Zone 2 migration and its development

In our study of the movement of dye markings over the PT we have confirmed the findings of Litton[6] and Alberti[7] that migration in this region takes a centrifugal direction. Our observations, carried out with modern fiberoptic equipment show outward movement of dye from the edge of the HM region below, and from the edge of the PF region above, to be the sole pattern of migration on the PT.

This pattern of zone 2 migration is in accordance with our observation of the development of zone 2 as the medial, proximal portion of the MP growing away from the fundus of the primary canal, including the narrower, upper wider area later covering the PF and the downward plunging 'tongue' of fundal epithelium later covering the HM. Zone 2 grows in early development into zone 3, which merges with zone 4, and this pathway of growth movement strongly suggests a life-long flux of epithelium away from the PT into the derivative of zone 3, the deep external canal.

Zone 1 migration and its development

The pathway of zone 1 movement of dye that we found in our otoscopic observations indicates that the PF and the malleus handle-covering epithelium moves as a single entity. To explain zone 1 migration its developmental history as the forerunner of the whole eardrum epithelium may be relevant. We would suggest that migratory movement may be present in this zone 1 precursor epithelium before it has expanded into the meatal plate. A tongue of fundus epithelium, the precursor of the HM epithelium, also seems to be present early and may share this movement. When the meatal plate is formed subsequently along the edge of zone 1, migration commences outwards into the MP from the whole edge of zone 1 giving rise to the zone 2 radial pathway of the more mature eardrum and canal.

A generation center at the tip of the meatal plate

It was possible to understand better the origin of migration over the PT and deep ear canal by analysis of the development of the early mouse MP in which it was found that the tip of zone 3 was bulbous, actively mitotic and extended always for a short distance on to the zone 2 side of the MP. A similar appearance is also observed in human fetal ears. It seems possible from this appearance that the tip of zone 3 at the interface with zone 2 functions as a generation center for the movement of zone 3 towards zone 4 from its earliest origin. This has been also suggested in the mature ear from experimental observations using the tritiated thymidine labeling technique[11,12]. The finding of a thickened and mitotically active zone 3 at its junction with zone 2 in both mouse and human would also imply that this region of zone 3 may be responsible for the movement of zone 2. The direction of movement, zone 2 to zone 3, would not, however, support a 'pushing' activity, but rather a 'pulling' one, for this flux.

From an early stage in the development of the MP, zone 2 appears thin and its cells become progressively attenuated. The suggestion that the marked activity of the zone 3 tip region represents an attraction for the cells of zone 2 is supported by the genesis of zone 2 in the mouse embryo only after zone 3 cells have formed, and the progressive thinning of zone 2 with the growth of the zone 3. The flow of zone 3 cells away from zone 2 may create a state of negative contact inhibition[13] in the zone 2 cells immediately adjacent, which could lead to the flow of these cells towards zone 3. The process could spread then across the whole of zone 2. An additional mitotic activity, albeit small in amount, would need to be postulated in zone 2 to replace the cells which have moved into zone 3.

References

1. Michaels L: An epidermoid formation in the developing middle ear: possible source of cholesteatoma. J Otolaryngol 15: 169–174, 1986

2. Wang RG, Hawke M, Kwok P: The epidermoid formation (Michaels' structure) in the developing middle ear. J Otolaryngol 16: 327–330, 1987

3. Michaels L: Origin of congenital cholesteatoma from a normally occurring epidermoid rest in the developing middle ear. Int J Ped Otolaryngol 15: 51–65, 1988

4. Levenson MJ, Michaels L, Parisier SC: Congenital cholesteatomas of the middle ear in children: origin and management. Otolaryngol Clin N Amer 22: 941–954, 1989

5. Stinson WD: Reparative processes in the membrana tympani. Arch Otolaryngol 24: 600–605, 1936

6. Litton WB: Epithelial migration over the tympanic membrane and external canal. Arch Otolaryngol 77: 254–257, 1963

7. Alberti PW: Epithelial migration on the tympanic membrane. J Laryngol Otol 74: 808–830, 1964

8. Michaels L, Soucek S: Auditory epithelial migration on the human tympanic membrane. II. The existence of two discrete migratory pathways and their embryologic correlates. Am J Anat 189: 189–200

9. Michaels L, Soucek S: Development of the stratified squamous epithelium of the human tympanic membrane and external canal: the origin of auditory epithelial migration. Am J Anat 184: 334–344, 1989

10. Hammar JA: Studien über die Entwicklung des Vorderdarms und einiger angrenzenden Organe. Arch Mikr Anat 59: 471–628, 1902

11. Litton WB: Epithelial migration in the ear: the location and characteristics of the generation center revealed by utilizing a radioactive desoxyribose nucleic acid precursor. Acta Oto-laryngol suppl 240: 1–37, 1968

12. Boedts D, Kuijpers W: Epithelial migration on the tympanic membrane. An experimental study. Acta Otolaryngol 85: 248–252, 1978

13. Lackie JM: *Cell Movement and Cell Behaviour*, pp 254–276. London: Allen and Unwin 1986

THE TYMPANIC AND MEATAL ANNULAR KERATINIZING EPITHELIUM

D. BOEDTS[1*] and D. BROEKAERT[2]

[1]ENT Department, UIA, University of Antwerp, B-2610 Wilrijk; [2]Laboratory of Physiological Chemistry, RUG, State University of Ghent, B-9000 Ghent; Belgium

For years the extraordinary proliferative and migratory capacity of the drumhead and adjacent bony canal epithelium has been noticed, the most striking example being the centripetal epithelial immigration towards the middle ear cleft in cholesteatoma pathology.

These properties are also expressed in the pathophysiology of closing tympanic perforations. Histological and clinical observations indicate that the healing of a tympanic membrane differs from the normal healing process of a skin wound where the squamous epithelium can migrate over a newly formed granulation tissue layer.

In a tympanic perforation, where there is no such underlying tissue, the healing of the connective tissue defect has a tendency to lag behind the healing of the epithelial layer. The very proliferative squamous tympanic epithelium spreads over the perforation, creating a typical appearance like a 'snake head' and tries before the connective tissue layer to close the gap[1,2] (Fig. 1).

So, tympanic perforations, even large ones, are frequently covered by a thin 'replacement membrane', consisting of a lateral squamous epithelial and a medial mucosal lining with in between remnants of a lamina propria, no more than $2-3$ μm thick, without fibroblasts, just enough to satisfy the vascular needs of epithelium and mucosal lining.

In these cases the very typical proliferative epithelial basal cells seem to be lacking, confirming the thesis that the upper epithelial layers are not generated by *in situ* proliferation, but that they have migrated from the periphery[3].

The proliferative capacity of the annular tympanic and bony wall epithelium is once more noticed in tympanoplasty surgery. It has been demonstrated that tympanic grafting material in any way acts as a scaffold. In the course of days and weeks the ear surgeon can observe the centripetal epithelial spreading over the graft which is of uppermost importance for the success of the operation.

Indeed, a race occurs between the epithelial migration on the one hand and the tendency to fibrosis or necrosis on the graft on the other[4] (Fig. 2).

According to autoradiographic experiments in animal drumheads the mitotic activity of the tympanic epithelium seems to be quite low under normal circumstances, and is mainly confined to the lower annular region[1,5] (Fig. 3).

McMinn and Taylor[6] could also observe only 26 mitotic figures in more than 20,000 epithelial cell controls in their guinea-pig drumhead experiments.

Under pathological conditions, however, the proliferative capacity of this epithelium becomes important and even large defects are covered in a relatively small period of time[1].

* *Correspondence to*: D. Boedts, Beukendreef 13, B-9831 Latem, Belgium

Middle Ear Structure, Organogenesis and Congenital Defects, pp. 57–62
edited by B. Ars and P. van Cauwenberge
©*1991 Kugler Publications, Amsterdam, New York*

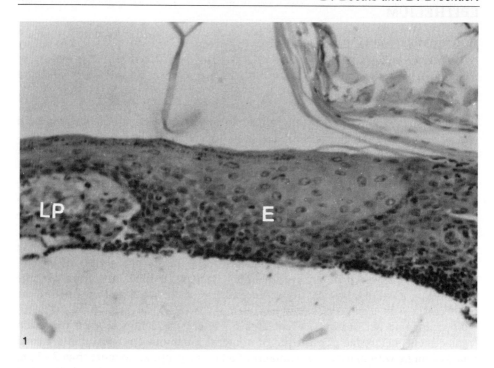

Fig. 1. Closing tympanic perforation. Squamous tympanic epithelium (E) spreads over the perforation LP: lamina propria (× 180).

Sakai *et al.*[7] and especially Proops, Boxall and co-authors[8-10] observed in their remarkable *in vitro* tissue culture studies a unique property of locomotion of the epidermal cells of the drumhead and adjacent bony auditory canal.

The 'mass movement' of these cells, also observed in cholesteatoma samples, was never noticed in normal extraconchal skin.

This streaming phenomenon of what they called 'the migratory skin' emanated from the inferior extremities of the drumhead and adjacent canal wall epithelium. There was no evidence of migration in the upper half and upper periphery of the tympanic membrane. This coincides remarkably with the localization of H^3 thymidine labels in the abovementioned autoradiographic experiments.

Research on the structure of the tympanic epithelium in the course of fetal and postnatal growth by Michaels and co authors[11] gives also evidence of the proliferative nature of the inferior annular region.

According to these authors (see also pp. 49 and following), three zones can be distinguished in the embryonic development of the stratified squamous epithelium of the tympanic membrane and external canal.

After opening of the meatal plate, zone 1 covers the pars flaccida, a tongue-shaped area passing inferiorly from it and a part of the postero-superior deep canal adjacent to it, zone 2 covers the pars tensa and zone 3 most of the deep external canal. According to Michaels proliferative activity, as indicated by a thickened epithelium, with rete ridges in later fetal life should be present in zone 1 and mainly in zone 3.

The existence of rete ridges, a localized thickening of the nucleated cell layers with

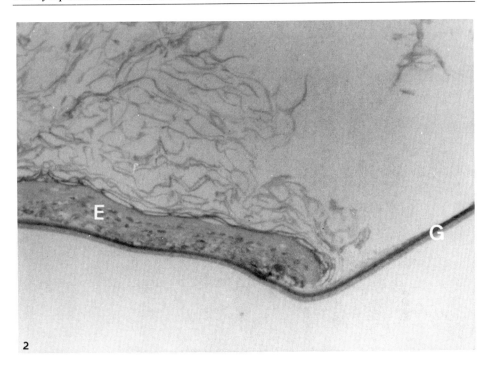

Fig. 2. Squamous tympanic epithelium (E) covering a graft (G) (× 30).

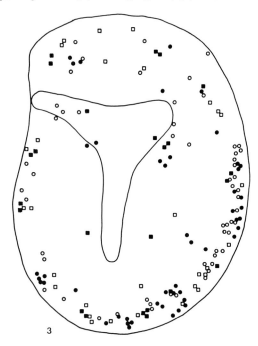

Fig. 3. Localization of H³-IDU labels in the tympanic epithelium in mice, two hours (○), two (●), four (□) and eight days (■) after injection of the isotope. Widespread labelling, with heaviest labelling near the lower annular region.

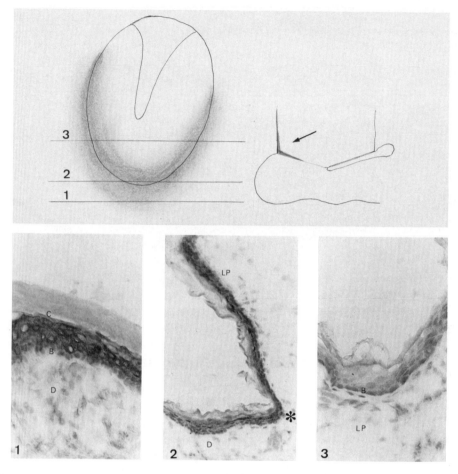

Fig. 4. Immunohistochemical staining for CK[16] via MoAb LL026. CK[16] mainly localized in the inferior deep meatal and annular epithelium.

1. Deep inferior meatal region. Marked staining of the suprabasal epithelial cell layers. D: dermis, B: stratum basale, C: stratum corneum ($\times$ 385).

2. Tympano-meatal angle (*). Significant staining on both meatal and tympanic sides. D: dermis, LP: lamina propria ($\times$ 240).

3. Section more centrally through pars tensa where the staining becomes weak. B: stratum basale, LP: lamina propria ($\times$ 385). (Reduction 40%).

flat basement membrane, has been confirmed in adult post-mortem observations, by Johnson *et al.*[12] at the lower deep meatal region, which corresponds with zone 3 mentioned by Michaels.

Recently, Broekaert *et al.*[13] in an immunohistochemical investigation of the cytokeratin expression of the squamous tympanic epithelium could undoubtedly demonstrate in humans the unusual proliferative nature of the lower annular region. Thus they noticed the unexpected appearance of CK_{16}, a hyperproliferative marker, known to have a limited distribution in healthy epidermis, in the deep inferior meatal and annular epithelium but not in the region of the umbo or pars flaccida (Fig. 4).

Cholesteatoma specimens also recurrently expressed CK_{16} in the suprabasal layers. These CK expression data argue for an intimate relationship between cholesteatoma pathology well known for their proliferative nature and the lower annular epidermal tissues.

For over a century a migrational phenomenon on the surface of the drumhead has been noticed in humans. Ink marks at various locations on the tympanic membrane present a centrifugal migration in the course of weeks. There is evidence that the centrifugal pattern is a movement of the superficial layers and that probably the stratum corneum acts as a passive flexible sheet and is transported on the underlying cells.

According to the 'marbles on a plate' hypothesis of Alberti[14] at random insertions of new corneocytes into the youngest corneocyte layer causes dislocation and sideways spread of the outermost keratin layers, from the bottom of the funnel formed by the drumhead, and adjacent bony auditory canal. So one should preferably use the term 'keratin dispersion', rather than 'migration'.

The physiological centrifugal keratin dispersion on the one hand and the proliferative and especially in pathological conditions migrational properties of the inferior annular region on the other, seem to be two distinct and different phenomena which both have clinical implications.

The keratin dispersion is a unique finely regulated physiological mechanism, well adapted to the necessity of cleaning the ear cavity and removal of foreign bodies and keratin.

Ear surgeons have, in the course of years, empirically noticed the importance of a meticulous and gently dissection and preservation of the annular epithelial lining for the success of their surgery. Absence of deep meatal and annular epithelium, *e.g.*, in cases of chronic granulomatous myringitis, remains an annoying otological problem.

The use of extraconchal 'non migratory' skin flaps is rarely successful. The same phenomenon can be observed in surgery for congenital middle ear malformations. According to the classification proposed by Marquet in 1971[15] essentially two types of atresia can be observed (see pp. 85 and following).

In type 1 atresia, when remnants of deep meatal skin remain, which are stripped and replaced during surgery, covering even partially the graft, no problems of skin migration occur, or only rarely so.

On the other hand, in the majority of the atresia type II cases, where a full-thickness extraconchal 'non-migratory' skin flap has to be used to cover the tympanic graft, epithelial migration is often delayed or even stops and granulation formation will appear in the depth of the graft which may lead to a stenotic ring and even a complete stenotic membrane.

The unique migratory possibilities of this annular and deep meatal epithelium can be used in unilateral epithelialization problems.

Thus, small free skin grafts from the contralateral healthy annular region of the same patient will quickly proliferate and migrate to cover the mesenchymal layer and are far more convenient than the usual full- or split-thickness extraconchal skin grafts.

As mentioned, suprabasal CK_{16} expression argues for an intimate relationship and provides biochemical evidence for the hyperproliferative nature of both the cholesteatoma matrix and the annular squamous epithelium.

The information and conclusions, gained from tissue culture experiments, immunohistochemical research, as well as embryological observations, all confirm the already for years clinically observed proliferative properties of the lower tympanic and mainly annular squamous epithelium. However, under normal conditions the mitotic activity of this epithelium seems to be quite low.

It is postulated that these proliferative and migratory phenomena only occur under pathological conditions, *e.g.*, in cases of perforations and cholesteatoma pathology, in tympanoplasty surgery where a centripetal movement is observed.

The question also arises whether this 'pathological' centripetal epithelial cell migration has not to be differentiated from the 'physiological' centrifugal keratin dispersion on top of the drumhead.

References

1. Reynen CJH, Kuypers W: The healing pattern of the drum membrane. Acta Otolaryngol (Stockh) Suppl 287: 1971
2. Boedts D, Ars B: Histopathological research on eardrum perforations. Arch Oto-Rhino-Laryngol 215: 55–59, 1977
3. Govaerts PJ, Jacob WA, Marquet J: Histological study of the thin replacement membrane of human tympanic membrane perforations. Acta Otolaryngol (Stockh) 105: 297–302, 1988
4. Boedts D: The behaviour of the keratinizing epithelium in tympanoplasty. J Laryngol Otol 98: 847–852, 1984
5. Boedts D: The tympanic epithelium in normal and pathological conditions. Acta Otorhinolaryngol (Belg) 32: 295–420, 1978
6. McMinn RMH, Taylor M: The cytology of repair in experimental perforations of the tympanic membrane. Br J Surg 53: 222–232, 1966
7. Sakai M, Miyake H, Shinkawa A: Tissue culture studies on the migratory property of cholesteatomas and external ear canal skin. In: *Cholesteatoma and Mastoid Surgery*, Proc 2nd Intern Conf. pp 153–160. Sadé J (ed). Amsterdam: Kugler Publ 1982
8. Proops D, Hawke M, Parkinson EK: Tissue culture of migratory skin of the external ear and cholesteatoma: a new research tool. J Otolaryngol 13(2): 63–69, 1984
9. Boxall JD, Proops DW, Michaels L: The specific locomotive activity of tympanic membrane and cholesteatoma epithelium in tissue culture. J Otolaryngol 17(4): 140–144, 1988
10. Boxall JD, Proops DW, Michaels K: Scanning electron microscopy of tympanic membrane epithelium during in vitro migration. J Otolaryngol 19: 57–61, 1990
11. Michaels L, Soucek S: Development of migrating epithelium on the tympanic membrane and external canal: the origin of auditory epithelial migration. Am J Anat 184: 334–344, 1989
12. Johnson A, Hawke M, Berger G: Surface wrinkles, cell ridges and desquamation in the external auditory canal. J Otolaryngol 13: 345–354, 1984
13. Broekaert D, Coucke P, Boedts D, Leperque S, Ramaekers F, Van Muyen G, Leigh I, Lane B, de Bersaques J, Marquet J: Cytokeratin expression in epidermal tissues, tympanic membrane and middle ear cholesteatoma, investigated with selective monoclonal antibodies. Ann Otolaryngol, in press.
14. Alberti PW: Epithelial migration on the tympanic membrane. J Laryngol Otol 78: 808–830, 1964
15. Marquet JF: Congenital malformations and middle ear surgery. J Roy Soc Med 74: 119–128, 1981

CHARACTERISTICS OF THE EMBRYONIC CONNECTIVE TISSUE IN THE MIDDLE EAR CLEFT

M. BERNAL-SPREKELSEN*, D. HOCH and H. HILDMANN

ENT-Department, University of Bochum, St. Elisabeth-Hospital (Head: Prof. Dr. H. Hildmann), 4630 Bochum, BRD

1. Introduction

The different roles attributed to the embryonic connective tissue (ECT) during the pneumatization of the middle ear cleft may be consulted in Hammar's, Wittmaack's, and others' publications.

In 1858, von Tröltsch[1] found ECT in the middle ear cleft of newborns. In the last century, this fact had medico-legal implications as it served to determine whether a child had been alive or not after birth, as no lumen ('air') was expected in the middle ear spaces during pregnancy. Air was supposed to 'invade' the middle ear as soon as breathing had started. In 1891, Hoffmann[2] proposed to take a tissue sample from the middle ear instead of the lung from children who had died to verify whether there had been breathing in the early perinatal period or not.

Bezold[3] and Wittmaack[4] suggested that the persistence of this mesenchyme could be related to the pathogenesis of primary cholesteatoma. Their theory on the retraction of the pars flaccida as a first step of cholesteatoma was accepted by Schwarz[5] and Steurer[6].

In 1929 Steurer[6] described rests of embryonic connective tissue in temporal bones of different ages.

Schwarz[7] observed the persistence of a myxomatous tissue in Prussak's space in 43% of newborns and in nearly 66% of cases with cholesteatoma in adults, mainly in the epitympanon. This tissue is believed to play a role in the pathogenesis of the cholesteatoma as the perimatrix, supporting the theory on the pathogenesis of cholesteatoma by means of papillary deep growth.

Although the mesenchyme has been described extensively before, no cellular measurements have been performed. To elucidate histological and cytological characteristics of the embryonic connective tissue we selected the perimalleolar region, where malleus, incus, and the chorda tympani served for regular anatomical orientation. It was our purpose to control the dynamics of the ECT in this area and to discuss the results with the observations of the literature.

2. Material and methods

More than 650 sections of 87 temporal bones aged four to seven months were studied histologically. The fetal age was confirmed by the biparietal diameter, a procedure which is commonly accepted[8]. Eight temporal bones aged four to five

* *Correspondence to*: Dr. M. Bernal-Sprekelsen, Am alten Stadtpark 47, 4630 Bochum 1, BRD

Middle Ear Structure, Organogenesis and Congenital Defects, pp. 63–68
edited by B. Ars and P. van Cauwenberge
©*1991 Kugler Publications, Amsterdam, New York*

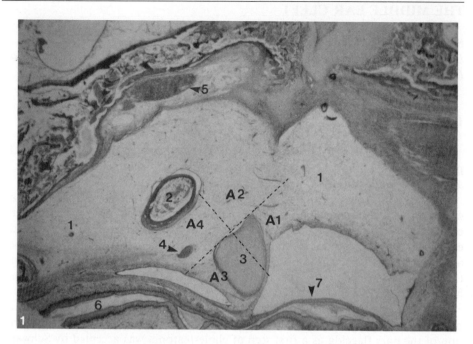

Fig. 1. Section of a temporal bone aged five to six months (No.1617; biparietal diameter = 5.5 cm). HE, magn. × 12.5, 75 μm ECT (1) occupying the tympanic cavity and surrounding the incus (2) and the malleus (3) completely. The presence of the chorda tympani (4) reveals that the section lays towards Prussak's space. Part of the facial nerve (5), the external ear canal (6) and the tympanic membrane (7) are visible. Division of the perimalleolar region into areas A1–A4 is marked by two imaginary lines (reduction 35%).

months, 32 aged six months, and 23 aged seven months (total n = 63) were used for morphometric measurements to determine the cell density of the perimalleolar ECT.

The sections of the temporal bones were performed from postero-superior to antero-inferior, not being exactly vertical.

A vertical line to the tympanic membrane crossing the malleus and a tangent on the superior margin of the malleus (Fig. 1) divided the perimalleolar region into four areas. Areas 1 and 3 were situated towards the tympanic membrane, covered by the mucosal lining. Areas 2 and 4 were located towards the epitympanon, without reaching it.

Morphometric measurements were performed microscopically with measuring lenses under a magnification of 40 ×, with the resulting area of 25 μm^2 to be counted.

Statistical evaluation was based on the comparison of the mean values.

Results

The ECT nearly filled up the tympanic cavity, surrounding the ossicles (Fig. 1) up to the epitympanon. The myxomatous tissue was rich in fibroblasts and interstitial substance. Mastocytes could be seen. Small capillaries crossed the tissue. A higher

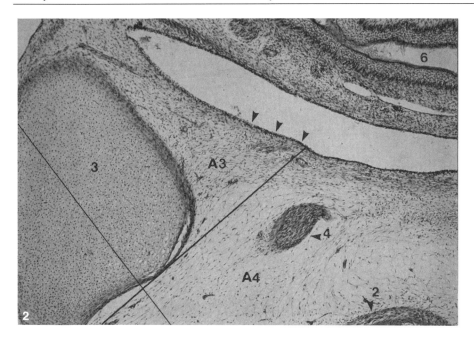

Fig. 2. Same section as Fig. 1. Area 3 (A3) under higher magnification ($\times$ 50), 80 μm. A higher cellular density is to be noticed towards the mucosa lining (arrows), getting lower towards the incus (2) (reduction 35%).

cellular density was observed towards the tympanic membrane (Figs. 2 and 3).

No histological differences were seen between specimens aged four months and those aged six or seven as far as the ECT is concerned.

The mean values of cellular density of each area revealed a higher density in areas 1 and 3 and a lower density in areas 2 and 4. Measurements gave evidence of a statistically significant difference ($p < 0,05$) between the mean values of the cell density of areas 1/3 and areas 2/4. The comparison of each single area showed that there were no changes in cellular density throughout time, that is, from the fourth to the seventh month (Fig. 4), with a statistical significance.

4. Discussion

Wittmaack[9] observed that the closure of the aditus ad antrum by connective tissue led to a reduced or bad pneumatization of the mastoid. Schwarz[5] often observed the persistence of embryonic connective tissue in the epitympanon of children with a bad pneumatization. The resorption of this tissue would lead to a retraction of the pars flaccida. According to Lange[10] and Steurer[6] these cushions of connective tissue resulted from inflammation.

Recently, Rauchfuss[11] attributed flat curves after tympanometric impedance, with conductive hearing loss and loss of stapedial reflex, to the persistence of embryonic tissue observed in the middle ear cavity of children aged up to one year.

As mentioned above, the ECT may persist after birth. At that time, its resorption

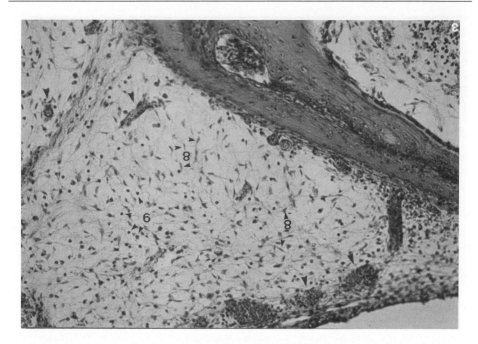

Fig. 3. Section of a temporal bone aged seven months (No.: 513/240; biparietal diameter = 7 cm), HE, × 125, 75 μm. Magnification of area 3. Histological structure of the ECT reveals fibroblasts (8, small arrows), mastocytes (9, small arrows) with interstitial spaces, and capillaries (arrows). The fibroblasts display a certain parallelism to the mucosa lining, being disposed more irregularly towards the incus (not shown) and the malleus (3) (reduction 35%).

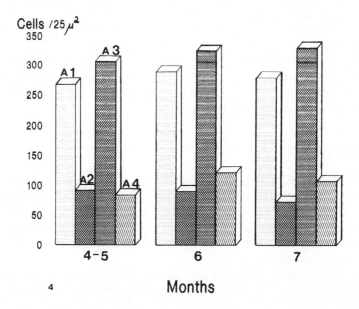

Fig. 4. Mean values of the cell density in areas 1−4 (A1−A4) in temporal bones, aged four to five, six and seven months.

may be completed or not. According to our results, the resorption does not occur before the seventh fetal month. While the cells display a remarkable uniformity, we believe that the interstitial substance is first resorbed, whereas the cells are supposed to become part of the inner layers of the middle ear cleft, being resorbed later on.

No epithelial elements were observed in 87 temporal bones. Therefore, genesis of cholesteatoma by means of epithelial cell sprinkling, as proposed by Cruveilhier[12] and Körner[13], is restricted to a few cases.

In 87 temporal bones individual variations of the ECT could not be observed. This is in contrast to the observations of Rüedi, who examined ten specimens up to seven months[14]. A differentiation of temporal bones into different types, as postulated by Rüedi, might occur later. Our results suggest that larger numbers of temporal bones are necessary to support Rüedi's theory. The pneumatization of the middle ear cleft due to resorption of the ECT described by Schwarz[15] and others has not been observed in our specimens. The middle ear clefts were occupied by ECT up to the seventh fetal month. The resorption of ECT seems to occur later. Older specimens have therefore to be studied.

Experimental data seem to support the possibility of cholesteatoma formation by means of papillary deep growth by formation of rete pegs: foreign bodies or substances in the external ear canal gave rise to cholesteatoma, as demonstrated by Berberich[16], Schröer[17], Rüedi[14], Grüninger[18], Bayer[19] and others. The so-called 'cutisstreifen' is able to develop papillary immigration even without stimulus, according to Link[20]. Infection of persistent ECT near the pars flaccida may allow papillary deep growth as proposed by Manasse[21], Schwarz[5,7], Lange[10], Rüedi[14] and others, the ECT being considered as perimatrix[5,7].

The persistence of ECT in Prussak's space has been related to the development of cholesteatoma, as its inflammation may lead to a retraction of the pars flaccida[3,4,6,7,22]. The retraction of the pars flaccida occurs quite often and in daily practice many epitympanic retractions may be observed, although not every retraction ends up in a cholesteatoma. The development of a cholesteatoma seems to require supplementary factors, such as a patulous tube, a pathologic middle ear gas exchange or middle ear infections, which may lead to a reactive proliferation tissue, as described in chronic otitis media, or to a perforation of the pars flaccida.

5. Conclusions

Eighty-seven temporal bones of fetuses aged four to seven months were studied histologically. Cellular measurements of the perimalleolar region showed that from the fourth to the seventh fetal month the embryonic connective tissue does not change: the cell density showed a remarkable uniformity between specimens of the same stage of development and between the different stages of development. The resorption of the ECT is therefore necessarily believed to occur later than described until now.

Our observations on the uniformity in the development of ECT are in contrast to Rüedi's theory on individual variations up to the seventh fetal month. The persistent ECT in Prussak's space and the epitympanon stimulates the discussion of the genesis of cholesteatoma.

References

1. Von Tröltsch cited in: Schwartze H: *Die Entwicklung der Ohrenheilkunde im letzten Decennium.* Arch Ohrenheilk 1, Vol 1, Würzburg 1864
2. Von Hoffmann E: *Lehrbuch der gerichtlichen Medizin.* Vienna: Urban und Schwarzenberg 1891
3. Bezold M: Cholesteatom, Perforation der Membrana flaccida und Tubenverschluß. Z Ohrenheilk 20: 5–28, 1890
4. Wittmaack K: Cholesteatombildung, Pneumatisation und Pneumatisationslehre. Arch Ohr-, Nasen-Kehlkopfheilk 125: 218–234, 1930
5. Schwarz M: Das individuelle Verhalten der Schleimhaut-propria im Mittelohr in ihrer Entwicklung und ihrem Gewebsaufbau. Z Hals-, Nasen-Ohrenheilk 289: 98–114, 1931
6. Steurer O: Schwierigkeiten bei der Diagnose der von der Shrapnellschen Membran ausgehenden Cholesteatome. HNO 2: 42, 1950
7. Schwarz M: *Das Cholesteatom im Mittelohr und im Gehörgang.* Stuttgart: Thieme 1966
8. Schmidt-Matthiesen H: *Gynäkologie und Geburtshilfe.* New York, Stuttgart: Schattauer Verlag 1985
9. Wittmaack K: Über die normale und pathologische Pneumatisation des Schläfenbeines. Jena: Gustav Fischer Verlag 1918
10. Lange W: Über die Entstehung der Mittelohr-cholesteatome. Z Hals-Nasen-Ohrenheilk 11: 250–271, 1925
11. Rauchfuss A: Die myxomatösen Reste im menschlichen Mittelohr. Laryngol Rhinol Otol 64: 243–248, 1985
12. Cruveilhier JC: *Anatomie pathologique du Corps humain.* Part II, 1828
13. Körner L: cited by Portmann C, Portmann M, Claverie G: *The Surgery of Deafness.* Valetta, Malta: Progress Press 1964
14. Rüedi L: Die Mittelohrraumentwicklung vom 5. Embryonalmonat bis zum 10. Lebensjahr. Acta Oto-laryngol Suppl 22, 1937
15. Schwarz M: *Die Schleimhäute des Ohres und der Luftwege. Biologie und Klinik.* Berlin, Göttingen, Heidelberg: Springer Verlag 1949
16. Berberich J: Das Mittelohrcholesteatom. Experimentelle und pathologisch-anatomische Untersuchungen. Hals-Nasen-Ohrenheilk 26: 1, 1927
17. Schröer R: Entwicklungsgeschichtliche und experimentelle Untersuchungen zur Genese der Mittelohrcholesteatome. Arch Ohr-Nasen-Kehlkopfheilk 170: 265, 1957
18. Grüninger G: *Über den Einfluß von Reizsubstanzen auf das Plattenepithel des äußeren Gehörganges und des Trommelfelles beim Kaninchen.* Academical Thesis, Tübingen 1977
19. Bayer J: *Über den Einfluß der experimentellen Otitis externa auf die Entstehung des Cholesteatoms.* Academical Thesis, Tübingen 1976
20. Link R: Die Bedeutung des Cutisstreifens bei der Entwicklung eines Mittelohrcholesteatoms. Acta Oto-laryngol (Stockholm) 49: 411, 1958
21. Manasse P: *Handbuch der Pathologischen Anatomie des Menschlichen Ohres.* Wiesbaden: JF Bergmann Verlag 1917
22. Schwarz M: Die Einsenkung der Shrapnellmembran. Arch Ohrenheilk 131: 16, 1932

INTERMEDIATE FILAMENT PROTEINS
Cell-type specific markers in differentiation, organogenesis and congenital pathology

DANIËL BROEKAERT*

Laboratory of Physiological Chemistry, State University of Ghent, K.L. Ledeganckstraat 35, B-9000 Ghent, Belgium

Introduction

In the last decade, our knowledge of the organization and function of the cytoplasm of higher eukaryotic cells has greatly expanded and it really has become impossible to cover the whole area of the cytoskeleton in a brief review. Currently, most excitement in studying the cytoskeleton is due to the realization that this structure provides significant information about the cellular origin and state of differentiation. This encourages the further exploration of these markers in normal cells and tissues, as well as under pathological conditions. Thus, this field is developing towards a form of molecular histology and histopathology, on the condition that cell biologists, biochemists, molecular biologists and pathologists mutually communicate.

This paper highlights the most widely accepted ideas and principles in the field of the cytoskeleton, concerning the intermediate filaments (IF) and the cytokeratin (CK) polypeptides in particular. It also focuses on certain applications and observations made in the field of middle ear congenital pathology, which in comparison with other domains, however, are not yet numerous. We regularly refer the reader to excellent reviews which can be consulted for primary references.

1. Cytoskeleton

It is now commonly accepted that elements belonging to the cytoskeleton are responsible for cell movement as well as movement within cells. Other fundamental functions associated with the cytoskeleton are adhesive interactions (cell-matrix and cell-cell interactions), cell division and possibly the transfer of 'information' from the plasma membrane to the nucleus, thereby affecting gene expression. Cytoskeletal structures − although responsible for cellular architecture − are not static but dynamic, *i.e.*, they are in a process of continuous assembly and disassembly.

The three major cytoskeletal networks are: (1) the microtubules, 25 nm in diameter; (2) the microfilaments, about 7 nm in diameter; (3) the intermediate filaments (IF), 10 nm in diameter (discussed in Section 2.). The microtrabecular lattice is sometimes discussed as a fourth filamentous network of the cytoskeleton. The biochemistry of microtrabeculae is however unknown and their existence itself remains an area of controversy.

---

* *Correspondence to:* D. Broekaert, at the above address.

Middle Ear Structure, Organogenesis and Congenital Defects, pp. 69–79
edited by B. Ars and P. van Cauwenberge
©*1991 Kugler Publications, Amsterdam, New York*

Microtubules represent highly-ordered polymers of the globular protein tubulin (native MW 110,000) and are composed of two similar subunits of 55,000, called the α- and β-chain. Of special interest are the polypeptides that co-purify with tubulin and promote the net polymerization *in vitro* (nucleation and elongation). Two major groups have been characterized. The first group has been designated MAPs or HMW polypeptides (microtubule-associated proteins of high molecular weight: MAP1: 340,000, MAP2: 270,000). The second group has been named 'tau' and is of low molecular weight (55,000−62,000). In interphase cells, microtubules traverse the cytoplasm over long distances, *i.e.*, from the nucleus to the plasma membrane where a specific interaction is postulated. The molecular mechanism of this interaction has not yet been fully clarified, but tubulin-like membrane proteins are postulated to be involved as a receptor and as an initiator of its polymerization.

Microtubuli are generally viewed as the supportive and less dynamic part of the cytoskeleton, constituted in different cell types from a narrow scope of molecules. This lack of selectivity has hampered their wide application in diagnostic pathology.

In addition, it has been realized that the cell membrane or at least the specialized structures involved in attachment of cytoplasmic filaments (*e.g.*, adhesion plaques) as well as those structures involved in cell-cell interactions (*e.g.*, gap junctions, desmosomes and tight junctions) are other major parts of the cytoskeleton. Desmoplakins, the major structural polypeptides of the desmosomal plaque are expressed in a highly conserved manner and are in addition to the cytokeratins (CKs) a particularly reliable marker of an epithelial origin used in diagnostic pathology. The only non-epithelial tissues expressing desmosomes and thus desmoplakins are the heart and meninges[1]. Furthermore, it has been recognized that the nuclear lamina inside the nuclear envelope is also involved in the cytoskeleton. Finally, the centrosomes that contribute to the organization of the cytoskeleton throughout cell division, remain during interphase as the center of microtubule organization. The existence of other organizing centers has been suggested, but has never been convincingly demonstrated.

In all cells, microfilaments result from the polymerization of the globular polypeptide actin (G-actin: 42 kD) to filaments (F-actin). Four muscle actins (two sarcomeric and two smooth muscle actins) and two non-muscle actins (β-, γ actin) have been characterized, suggesting some molecular diversification of the backbone polypeptide. All actins are characterized by the ability to interact with myosins. In addition, an increasing number of polypeptides have been found in various cells that interact with actin and influence its polymerization and/or depolymerization, its organization in filaments, its interaction with myosin or cause cross-linking of actin filaments. The best characterized of these associated polypeptides are tropomyosin, α-actinin, fragmin, villin, fimbrin, gelactins, filamin. Several lines of evidence suggest that microfilaments not only form cytoplasmic stress fibers but in addition can be associated directly or indirectly with the cell membrane, or even that they are a major component of the isolated plasma membrane (*e.g.*, in erythrocytes). It is frequently suggested that actin filaments belong to the dynamic (contractile) part of the cytoskeleton and function in the regulation of the deformability of the cell membrane. They represent part of the submembranous lattice that is anchored to the cell membrane via distinct polypeptides (*e.g.*, ankyrin and ankyrin-related polypeptides). The diversity of actin-associated proteins suggests that more than one molecular mechanism is involved in the integration of microfilaments within the cytoskeletal network. The still-increasing complexity and variability of the microfilament system in different cell types and under different conditions is certainly a major reason for the absence of a real break-through in histopathology. Nevertheless, monoclonal antibodies to various microfilamentous elements have been valuable tools to study the cellular cytoskeleton[2] and actin isoform typing was promising in differentiating certain smooth and striated muscular tumors[3, 4].

Additional information concerning the cytoskeletal architecture and the properties of the cytoskeletal elements may be found in many excellent review articles[1, 5–10].

2. Intermediate filaments

IF have been described in virtually all differentiated cell types of higher eukaryotics. The most widely discussed role for IF is that of an intracellular support (via the mechanical integration of various cytoplasmic organelles) and involvement in maintaining cell shape.

In contrast to microfilaments and microtubules where the backbones are composed of similar polypeptides in different cells, high-resolution biochemical and immunological techniques have distinguished five subclasses of α-helix rich polypeptides that constitute IF in different tissues or cells:

1. (Cyto)keratin or (CK) filaments or tonofilaments, found in all epithelial cells and cells of epithelial origin (discussed in Section 3).

2. Vimentin(decamin) filaments, found in mesenchymal cells and cells of mesenchymal origin. Vimentin has a molecular weight of 52,000.

3. Desmin (skeletin) filaments, observed in muscle cells, either smooth, skeletal or cardiac muscle cells. Desmin is a 50,000 kD polypeptide.

4. Neurofilaments (NF) which are characteristically present in neurons and are composed of three distinct polypeptides with molecular weight of 210,000, 160,000 and 68,000 (so-called neurofilament triplet).

5. Glial filaments, present in all cell types of glial origin (*e.g.*, astrocytes) and composed of the 50,000 glial filament acidic protein (GFAP).

These subclasses of IF are generally associated with particular cell types or cell lineages which enable them to be used diagnostically[11]. However, it has been recognized that some normal cell types *in vivo* as well as *in vitro* have more than one type of IF subunit (co-expression, recently reviewed[12, 13]). The growing list of exceptions and addenda to the principal rule of IF expression does however not jeopardize the usefulness of IF typing, but argues for a less dogmatic application of the biological and diagnostic significance of IF and the shift from a rigid histogenetic scheme to a more complex and dynamic interpretation. Far from depriving cell biologists of a primary tool however, this enables us to interpret unexpected findings and to take advantage of the complex expression patterns observed[13]. Recently, it has been stressed that IF expression should be modulated by the cellular microenvironment[13].

The tissue-specific expression of IF subclasses is (largely) retained during neoplastic transformation and no additional IF subclasses are expressed in neoplastic outgrowths[14, 16]. Nevertheless, certain neoplastic tissues tend to co-express different types of IF polypeptides[17, 18]. This applies not only to benign and malignant tumors arising from normal cells already committed to co-expression (*e.g.*, smooth muscle cells, mesothelial cells) but also to neoplastic cells which express *de novo* IF polypeptides not synthesized by the normal cell counterpart, in addition to the proper IF subclass[4, 13, 19], *e.g.*, certain metastatic tumor cells of epithelial origin that co-express vimentin next to CK filaments[20]. So, tumor diagnosis based on IF typing clearly requires a critical interpretation. When combined with the classic morphological analysis of tumor cells and additional clinical information however, IF typing can greatly refine the cytologic diagnosis and significantly decrease errors[21].

In the last decade, the field of IF has been explored by various approaches including molecular biological techniques, leading to deeper insights in, *e.g.*, the organization, complexity, evolution, divergence and chromosomal localization of IF genes. Based on nucleotide sequence data, a revised classification of IF was proposed, now classified into distinct sequence types (type I: acidic CKs; II: neutral-basic CKs; III: vimentin, desmin and GFAP; IV: NF triplet). Recently, a fifth sequence type (V) was included, referring to lamins (four polypeptides in the MW range of 60,000−70,000) which form the karyoskeleton along the inner surface of the eukaryotic nuclear membrane. Furthermore, the IF and macrofibril (self-)assembly via the two-chain coiled coil structures, the four-chain complexes (protofilaments) and the higher-order structures has been unravelled. We emphasize the reviews[14, 22−27] for detailed information.

3. Cytokeratin filaments

CK filaments are perhaps the most atypical of all IF subclasses. Combining all available data from high-resolution two-dimensional gel electrophoretic analysis of CK polypeptides, revealed a family of 19 different polypeptides (numbering and classification: see the CK catalog[28]). The CK molecular weights vary from 40,000−67,000 and the subunits fall into two distinct groups called subfamily B, *i.e.*, the neutral to basic CKs (also called type II CKs, CK1−8, 52−67 kD, pI 6−7.8) and subfamily A of the acidic CKs (also called type I CKs, CK9−19, 40−63 kD, pI 4.9−5.7). In addition, this subdivision has an immunological basis (presence of common determinants within each member of a subfamily) and is in accordance with the molecular biological approach (positive hybrid selection data by means of specific recombinant cDNA probes).

In various epithelia and under varying conditions, subsets of two to ten polypeptides with varying composition are expressed. The rules that govern the CK expression are summarized in the concept of the 'differential expression of CKs'. Thus, the CK composition of the subset expressed in the epidermis depends on the stage of embryological development, the localization of the epidermis, the stage of histological differentiation and keratinocyte maturation, the conditions of growth (*in vivo* as well as *in vitro*), the pathological conditions of cells and tissues inclusive of tumorous growth. Furthermore, the CK complement expressed depends on the histological type of the epithelium and on the cell type under consideration (*e.g.*, Merkel cells, myoepithelial cells).

It has also emerged from numerous investigations that coordinated doublets of an acidic and a basic CK polypeptide are preferentially expressed (the concept of 'CK pairs'). This reflects the straightforward mechanism of the IF assembly itself and the functional significance of each CK polypeptide. This second concept explains the observation that CK pairs are (obligatorily) formed between each member of the A subfamily and a corresponding member of the B subfamily and further implies that within each CK pair, the B member will be always larger than the A member by approximately 8 kD. In other words, the members of a CK pair follow similar rules of expression and occupy identical size ranks in each subfamily.

Apart from CK19, which is present in most of the non-epidermal epithelia and has no preferential partner, and CK11 and CK15 of which available data are actually sparse, the functional significance of the human CK pairs can be summarized as follows:
- CK1,2 (doublet) and CK10 are markers for phenotypic keratinization including cornification (*e.g.*, in the epidermis at the suprabasal level);
- CK3 and CK12 are among the most prominent CKs in the corneal epithelium and are cornea-specific;
- CK4 and CK13 are most prevalent in non-cornified stratified squamous epithelia of internal organs (*e.g.*, exocervix, esophagus);
- CK5 and CK14 are present in all stratified epithelia from the basal level onwards;
- CK6 and CK16 are typical for hyperproliferative or undifferentiated keratinocytes;
- CK7 and CK17 are molecular markers for simple and some complex (pseudo-) stratified (*e.g.*, glandular epithelia) and transitional epithelia;
- CK8 and CK18 are expressed mainly in simple and transitional epithelia, and in mesothelial cells.

The evidences supporting the above statements are described in more detail in many reviews[24, 26, 27, 29-31].

The functional significance of human CKs is reproduced with great fidelity under pathological conditions, even in epithelial neoplasms. This third rule provides another role for CK immunohistochemistry, namely to assist in subclassifications of carcinomas and to indicate whether a given tumor is more likely to be derived from a certain epithelium. Unfortunately, certain tumors do not strictly maintain the CK phenotype of their normal tissue counterpart, making CK typing ineffective in revealing the precise cell origin of these tumors[4, 11, 14, 28-30, 32].

4. Applications in middle ear congenital pathology

The achievements of the cytoskeletal research, summarized in the foregoing sections, have not yet been widely applied in otology-related research in general and middle ear organogenesis and congenital pathology in particular. One of the few topics in which a certain continuity has been reached — at least from a scientific point of view — is the organogenesis of the inner ear and the inner ear structures in newborn and adult humans and laboratory animals[33-46]. Unfortunately, studies on the human middle ear with regard to organogenesis have until now been lacking, although the field is ready for exploration. A first example with regard to congenital pathology is presented here. It is part of a wider goal, *i.e.*, to explore the true nature of middle ear cholesteatoma, by a systematic screening of the so-called keratinization markers.

Based on immunohistochemical CK typing, we and others have already explored the acquired middle ear cholesteatoma, a lesion of which the etiology and pathogenesis was unknown before and a current topic of debate[47−50]. The results obtained indicated an epidermal-type CK pattern in the cholesteatoma matrix. They further pointed to the locally hyperproliferative nature of the disease and to some focal or more extended disturbances of the terminal phase of keratinization. Combined CK data obtained on epithelia of deep meatus, tympanic membrane, middle ear mucosa and cholesteatoma matrix argue for an intimate relationship between aural cholesteatoma and epidermal tissues in the area. The mechanism(s) by which these epidermal epithelia become installed in the middle ear cavity have not however been traced.

In the meantime, the so-called primary or congenital cholesteatomas have been included in our investigations. It concerns the least frequent type, since most authors estimate that it represents less than 2% of the total amount of cholesteatoma lesions. Strictly speaking, this figure is an approximation, since the congenital origin of the lesions have been presumed but never determined for certain[51−56]. Congenital or developmental cholesteatomas occur behind a perfectly normal eardrum, mostly in children, without any previous otitis media or complaints of Eustachian tube dysfunction. They were subdivided by their location within the temporal bone (petrous pyramid, the mastoid and middle ear cleft[57, 58]). In the middle ear, they preferentially occur on the medial wall of the cavity and near the tympanic isthmus[59−61]. Since the tympanic isthmus is the junction of the first and second branchial arch, their origin could be linked to the inward migration of the external canal ectoderm into the middle ear, at the early stage of development. This suggests a developmental error, namely the absence of a stop-signal near the tympanic ring that contains the ectoderm at the annular plane[59, 60]. Thus, the etiology of the middle ear congenital lesions is essentially the awakening of an embryonic or ectodermal rest in the middle ear itself. Islands of stratified squamous epithelia, epidermoids and microkeratomas have indeed been found in middle ear mucosa of human embryos[60, 62, 63]. The expansion to clinically important lesions is however not documented. Furthermore, since it remains difficult to prove unequivocally that in these ears there were indeed expanding embryonic rests, some authors reject a congenital origin and refer to metaplasia of the middle ear mucosa due to inflammation, still others argue for multiple etiologies of lesions behind the tympanic membrane, including metaplasia[64, 65].

The precise mechanism underlying the origin of congenital cholesteatomas can also be revealed, at least partially, by CK immunotyping. The samples included in our study were selected with the utmost severity and were all obtained from children with a perfectly normal drum and without any history of tubal dysfunction and otitis media. The monoclonal antibody panel used has been discussed elsewhere and the method of choice was predominantly the indirect immunoperoxidase technique, applied on unfixed cryoslices[47−48]. Altogether, in addition to the mesenchymal marker vimentin, ten out of 19 CK polypeptides were individually screened, including prominent markers for stratified epithelia (CK5/14), and for stratified squamous epithelia, cornified and non-cornified (respectively CK10 and CK4/13). In addition, major markers for simple and pseudo-stratified epithelia (CK7, 8, 18, 19) and for hyperproliferative keratinocytes (CK16) were provided (see Section 3).

The results obtained (Table 1) point to the presence of CK5, 10, 14 and 16 in all lesions examined so far (n = 5). CK5, 10 and 14 were recurrently observed in an epidermal mode, _i.e._, CK5 and 14 were noticed from the basal cell layer onwards,

TABLE 1. Cytokeratin expression in congenital and acquired middle ear cholesteatoma, compared with epidermis and middle ear mucosa.

Cytokeratin	Middle ear cholesteatoma		Middle ear mucosa	Epidermis
	congenital	acquired		
CK4	−	−ᶠ	+	−
CK5	+	+	(+)	+
CK7	−	−ᶠ	+	−
CK8	−	−ᶠ	+	−
CK10	+	+	−	+
CK13	−	−ᶠ	−	−
CK14	+	+	+	+
CK16	+	+	−	−/+*
CK18	−	−ᶠ	+	−
CK19	−	−ᶠ	+	−

f : focally expressed (terminal keratinization)
* : site-specific expression, *i.e.*, deep meatus

while CK10 became a prominent marker of immediately suprabasal and terminal differentiation stages. In addition, a prominent staining of CK16 was obligatorily observed suprabasally. In three of the cases examined, the expression of the CK16 epitope irregularly persisted in the stratum corneum. Expression of CK4, 7, 8, 13, 18 and 19 − even in minor amounts − was never observed.

The conclusion from the above data is clear, *i.e.*, the so-called congenital cholesteatomas are committed to the same type of CK expression program as the acquired lesions[47-50]. They represent an epidermal-type CK set, completed with a major expression of CK16, pointing to the hyperproliferative nature of the lesion. Our combined positive and negative data do not favor a metaplastic origin from middle ear mucosa as the CK spectrum of the lesion does not contain any of the prominent markers of the recipient mucosa (*i.e.*, CK4, 7, 8, 18 and 19).

A squamous metaplastic lesion would be expected to express a complex CK set, composed of one or more of the major CKs from the recipient tissue, together with CKs representative of a cornified stratified squamous epithelium[66-67]. Instead of metaplasia, thus the awakening of an ectodermal rest, in the wrong place, seems to be in accordance with our CK data.

Conclusion

It may certainly be stated that in the last decade, highly conserved cytoskeletal polypeptides have become a reliable and independent marker for discovering cell-lineage and cellular differentiation. In addition to the great number of selective antibodies already available, new probes may in the near future complement the current panels of antibodies. Altogether, it furnishes a new molecular approach not only for diagnostic pathology but also for basic sciences like cytology, histology and embryology as well. At the same time, it is clear that the field has become increasingly complicated, mainly because of the numerous exceptions to the previously established rules and avoiding these pitfalls is another task for those concerned. In spite of the restricted applications in congenital pathology in animal models and humans, it is the conviction of those involved in the field that the use of cytoskeletal markers is a tremendous stride forward in the characterization of histogenetic defects.

A call is made for further application of these markers in studies dealing with middle ear organogenesis and congenital pathology, and to make up the arrears. The identity of developmental tumor-like anomalies of the middle ear (*e.g.*, hamartomas, salivary choristomas, glial masses[68]) may be easily confirmed by immunohistochemical staining using cytoskeletal polypeptides. Furthermore, a molecular approach of the embryology of the middle ear may be helpful to understand well the congenital malformations of the middle ear.

These middle ear anomalies include particular forms of atresia, microtia and deformed malleus and incus, referring to an arrest of the normal development from the first branchial groove and Meckel's cartilage, as well as cases of stapedial anomalies including fixation to the oval window, referring to a developmental error from the second branchial arch and Reichert's cartilage. Some of these anomalies are part of the well-known Treacher-Collins syndrome, Crouzon's disease and the Hunter-Hurler syndrome[69]. Now that the molecular tools are established, it becomes a major goal to unravel the developmental stage-dependent changes of the cytoskeleton during middle ear organogenesis and fine cytodifferentiation, whether normal or pathological. A study of the exact nature of the middle ear anomalies not only provides insight into the period of embryonic development when the deviating development occurred, but also indirectly suggests the other anomalies that might be encountered.

Acknowledgements

The author is indebted to Marc Davey for critical revision of the manuscript and to H. Eto, E.B. Lane, I. Leigh, F. Ramaekers and G. Van Muijen for their generous gifts of antibodies. The financial support of the Belgian Nationaal Fonds voor Wetenschappelijk Onderzoek is gratefully acknowledged.

References

1. Moll R, Cowin P, Kapprell H-P, Franke WW: Desmosomal proteins: new markers for identification and classification of tumors. Lab Invest 54: 4–25, 1986
2. Lin JJC, Feramisco JR, Blose SH, Matsumura F: Monoclonal antibodies to cytoskeletal proteins. In: *Monoclonal Antibodies and Functional Cell Lines*. Kennett RH, Bechtol KB, McKearn TJ (eds) New York: Plenum Publishing Corporation 1984
3. Schürch W, Skalli O, Seemayer TA, Gabbiani G: Intermediate filament proteins and actin isoforms as markers for soft tissue tumor differentiation and origin. I. Smooth muscle tumors. Am J Pathol 128: 91–103, 1987
4. Corwin DJ, Gown AM: Review of selected lineage-directed antibodies useful in routinely processed tissues. Arch Pathol Lab Med 113: 645–652, 1989
5. Weatherbee JA: Membranes and cell movement: interaction of membranes with the proteins of the cytoskeleton. Int Rev Cytol, Suppl 12: 113–176, 1981
6. Weber K, Osborn M: Cytoskeleton: definition, structure and gene regulation. Path Res Pract 175: 128–145, 1982

7. Geiger B: Membrane-cytoskeleton interaction. Biochim Biophys Acta 737: 305–341, 1983
8. McIntosh JR: The centrosome as an organizer of the cytoskeleton. In: *Modern Cell Biology*. McIntosh JR (ed). New York: Alan R Liss Inc 1983
9. Niggli V, Burger MM: Interaction of the cytoskeleton with the plasma membrane. J Membrane Biol 100: 97–121, 1987
10. French SW, Kawahara H, Katsuma Y, Ohta M, Swierenga SHH: Interaction of intermediate filaments with nuclear lamina and cell periphery. Electron Microsc Rev 2: 17–51, 1989
11. Nagle RB: Intermediate filaments. Efficacy in surgical pathologic diagnosis. Am J Clin Pathol 91(Suppl): S14–S18, 1989
12. Kasper M, Karsten U: Coexpression of cytokeratin and vimentin in Rathke's cysts of the human pituitary gland. Cell Tissue Res 253: 419–424, 1988
13. Coggi G, Dell'Orto P, Braidotti P, Coggi A, Viale G: Coexpression of intermediate filaments in normal and neoplastic human tissues: a reappraisal. Ultrastruct Pathol 13: 501–514, 1989
14. Osborn M, Weber K: Tumor diagnosis by intermediate filament typing: a novel tool for surgical pathology. Lab Invest 48: 372–394, 1983
15. Ramaekers FCS, Puts JJG, Moesker O, Kant A, Huysmans A, Haag D, Jap PHK, Herman CJ, Vooijs GP: Antibodies to intermediate filament proteins in the immunohistochemical identification of human tumors: an overview. Histochem J 15: 691–713, 1983
16. Roholl PJM, De Jong ASH, Ramaekers FCS: Application of markers in the diagnosis of soft tissue tumours. Histopathology 9: 1019–1035, 1985
17. Gown AM, Gabbiani G: Intermediate-sized (10 nm) filaments in human tumors. In: *Advances in Immunohistochemistry*. Masson Monographs in Diagnostic Pathology, Vol. 7. DeLellis RA (ed). New York: Masson Publishing USA Inc 1984
18. Ramaekers FCS, Vooijs GP, Huysmans ACLM, Salet-v.d. Pol MRJ, van Aspert-van Erp AJM, Beck HLM: Immunohistochemistry as an aid in diagnostic cytopathology. In: *Advances in Immunohistochemistry*. DeLellis RA (ed). New York: Raven Press 1988
19. Battifora H: Clinical applications of the immunohistochemistry of filamentous proteins. Am J Surg Pathol 12 (Suppl): 24–42, 1988
20. Putts JJG, Vooijs GP, Huysmans A, van Aspert A, Ramaekers FCS: Cytoskeletal proteins as tissue-specific markers in cytopathology. In: *Experimental Cell Biology*. Rüttner JR, Sherbet GV, Ramseier H, Helson L, Wolsky A (eds). Basel: Karger AG 1986
21. Domagala W, Lasota J, Chosia M, Szadowska A, Weber K, Osborn M: Diagnosis of major tumor categories in fine-needle aspirates is more accurate when light microscopy is combined with intermediate filament typing. Cancer 63: 504–517, 1989
22. Lazarides E: Intermediate filaments as mechanical integrators of cellular space. Nature 283: 249–256, 1980
23. Osborn M, Weber K: Intermediate filaments proteins: a multigene family distinguishing major cell lineages. Trends Biochem Sci 11: 469–472, 1986
24. Steinert PM, Steven AC, Roop DR: The molecular biology of intermediate filaments. Cell 42: 411–419, 1985
25. Geisler N, Weber K: Structural aspects of intermediate filaments. In: *Cell and Molecular Biology of the Cytoskeleton*. Shay JW (ed). New York: Plenum Publishing Corporation 1986
26. Roop DR, Steinert PM: The structure and evolution of intermediate filament genes. In: *Cell and Molecular Biology of the Cytoskeleton*. Shay JW (ed). New York: Plenum Publishing Corporation 1986
27. Steinert PM, Roop DR: Molecular and cellular biology of intermediate filaments. Ann Rev Biochem 57: 593–625, 1988
28. Moll R, Franke WW, Schiller DL, Geiger B, Krepler R: The catalog of human cytokeratins: patterns of expression in normal epithelia, tumors and cultured cells. Cell 31: 11–24, 1982
29. Sun T-T, Eichner R, Schermer A, Cooper D, Nelson WG, Weiss RA: Classification, expression, and possible mechanisms of evolution of mammalian epithelial keratins: A unifying model. In: *Cancer Cells 1, The Transformed Phenotype*. Levine AJ, Vande Woude GF, Topp WC, Watson JD (eds). Cold Spring Harbor Laboratory 1984
30. Cooper D, Schermer A, Sun T-T: Classification of human epithelia and their neoplasms using monoclonal antibodies to keratins: strategies, applications, and limitations. Lab Invest 52: 243–256, 1985
31. Fuchs E: Keratins as biochemical markers of epithelial differentiation. Trends in Genet 4: 277–281, 1988

32. Battifora H: The biology of the keratins and their diagnostic applications. In: *Advances in Immunohistochemistry*. DeLellis RA (ed) New York: Raven Press 1988
33. Flock A, Bretscher A, Weber K: Immunohistochemical localization of several cytoskeletal proteins in inner ear sensory and supporting cells. Hearing Res 6: 75–89, 1982
34. Thornell L-E, Anniko M, Virtanen I: Cytoskeletal organization of the human inner ear. I. Expression of intermediate filaments in vestibular organs. Acta Otolaryngol (Stockh) Suppl 437: 5–27, 1987
35. Anniko M, Thornell L-E, Virtanen I: Cytoskeletal organization of the human inner ear. II. Characterization of intermediate filaments in the cochlea. Acta Otolaryngol (Stockh) Suppl 437: 29–54, 1987
36. Thornell L-E, Anniko M: Cytoskeletal organization of the human inner ear. III. Expression of actin in the cochlea. Acta Otolaryngol (Stockh) Suppl 437: 55–63, 1987
37. Anniko M, Thornell L-E: Cytoskeletal organization of the human inner ear. IV. Expression of actin in vestibular organs. Acta Otolaryngol (Stockh) Suppl 437: 65–76, 1987
38. Anniko M, Thornell L-E, Ramaekers FCS, Stigbrand T: Cytokeratin diversity in epithelia of the human inner ear. Acta Otolaryngol (Stockh) 108: 385–396, 1989
39. Wikström SO, Anniko M, Thornell L-E, Virtanen I: Developmental stage-dependent pattern of inner ear expression of intermediate filaments. Acta Otolaryngol (Stockh) 106: 71–80, 1988
40. Anniko M, Sjöström B, Thornell L-E, Virtanen I: Cytoskeletal identification of intermediate filaments in the inner ear of the Jerker mouse mutant. Acta Otolaryngol (Stockh) 107: 191–201, 1989
41. Anniko M, Wenngren BI, Thornell L-E, Virtanen I: Expression of intermediate filament proteins in the inner ear of the Dancer mouse mutant. Acta Otolaryngol (Stockh) 108: 45–54, 1989
42. Anniko M, Thornell L-E, Hulterantz M, Virtanen I, Ramaekers FCS, Stigbrand T: Prenatal low-dose gamma irradiation of the inner ear induces changes in the expression of intermediate filaments. Acta Otolaryngol (Stockh) 108: 206–216, 1989
43. Schulte BA, Adams JC: Immunohistochemical localization of vimentin in the gerbil inner ear. J Histochem Cytochem 37: 1787–1797, 1989
44. Schrott A, Egg G, Spoendlin H: Intermediate filaments in the cochleas of normal and mutant (w/w^v, sl/sl^d) mice. Arch Otorhinolaryngol 245: 250–254, 1988
45. Kasper M, Stosiek P, Varga A, Karsten U: Immunohistochemical demonstration of the co-expression of vimentin and cytokeratin(s) in the guinea pig cochlea. Arch Otorhinolaryngol 244: 66–68, 1987
46. Anniko M, Thornell L-E, Gustavsson H, Virtanen I: Intermediate filaments in the newborn inner ear of the mouse. Otorhinolaryngology 48: 98–106, 1986
47. Broekaert D, Cornille A, Eto H, Leigh I, Ramaekers F, Van Muijen G, Coucke P, De Bersaques J, Kluyskens P, Gillis E: A comparative immunohistochemical study of cytokeratin and vimentin expression in middle ear mucosa and cholesteatoma, and in epidermis. Virchows Archiv A Pathol Anat 413: 39–51, 1988
48. Broekaert D, Coucke P, Boedts D, Leperque S, Ramaekers F, Van Muijen G, Leigh I, Lane B, De Bersaques J, Marquet J: Cytokeratin expression in epidermal tissues, tympanic membrane and middle ear cholesteatoma, investigated with selective monoclonal antibodies. In: Proceedings of the Conference on the Eustachian Tube and Middle Ear Diseases. Amsterdam/Milano: Kugler & Ghedini Publications 1990
49. Van Blitterswijk CA, Grote JJ: Cytokeratin expression in cholesteatoma matrix, meatal epidermis and middle ear epithelium. A preliminary report. Acta Otolaryngol (Stockh) 105: 529–532, 1988
50. Van Blitterswijk CA, Broekaert D, Lutgert MW, Grote JJ: Cytokeratin expression in relation to cholesteatoma pathogenesis. In: *Cholesteatoma and Mastoid Surgery*. Tos M, Thomsen J, Peitersen E (eds). Amsterdam/Milano: Kugler & Ghedini 1989
51. Schwartz RH, Grundfast KM, McAveney WJ, Merida MA, Feldman B: Congenital middle ear cholesteatoma. Am J Dis Child 137: 501–502, 1983
52. Schwartz RH, Grundfast KM, Feldman B, Linde RE, Hermansen KL: Cholesteatoma medial to an intact tympanic membrane in 34 young children. Pediatrics 74: 236–240, 1984
53. McDonald TJ, Cody DTR, Ryan RE: Congenital cholesteatoma of the ear. Ann Otol Rhinol Laryngol 93: 637–640, 1984
54. Alaminos D, Olaizola F, Rodriguez S, Prades J, Arroyo R: Cholesteatoma with intact tympanic membrane. Etiopathogenesis, clinical history and treatment. In: *Cholesteatoma and Mastoid Surgery*. Tos M, Thomsen J, Peitersen E (eds). Amsterdam/Milano: Kugler & Ghedini 1989
55. Ralli G, Magliulo G: The cholesteatoma behind an intact tympanic membrane: personal experiences. In: *Cholesteatoma and Mastoid Surgery*. Tos M, Thomsen J, Peitersen E (eds). Amsterdam/Milano: Kugler & Ghedini 1989

56. Radulovic RB, Opric MM, Krejovic BM, Bankovic SS: Some remarks on the pathogenesis of cholesteatoma. In: *Cholesteatoma and Mastoid Surgery*. Tos M, Thomsen J, Peitersen A (eds). Amsterdam/Milano: Kugler & Ghedini 1989
57. Derlacki EL, Clemis JD: Congenital cholesteatoma of the middle ear and mastoid. Ann Otol Rhinol Laryngol 74: 706–727, 1965
58. Peron DL, Schuknecht HF: Congenital cholesteatoma with other anomalies. Arch Otolaryngol 101: 498–505, 1975
59. Aimi K: Role of the tympanic ring in the pathogenesis of congenital cholesteatoma. Laryngoscope 93: 1140–1146, 1983
60. Aimi K: Embryogenesis of congenital cholesteatoma. In: *Cholesteatoma and Mastoid Surgery*. Tos M, Thomsen J, Peitersen E (eds). Amsterdam/Milano: Kugler & Ghedini 1989
61. Michaels L: Origin of congenital cholesteatoma from a normally occurring rest in the developing middle ear. Int J Pediat Otolaryngol 15: 51–65, 1988
62. Akaan-Pentillä E: Middle ear mucosa in newborn infants. A topographical and microanatomical study. Acta Otolaryngol (Stockh) 93: 251–259, 1982
63. Michaels L: An epidermoid formation in the developing middle ear: possible source of cholesteatoma. J Otolaryngol 15: 169–174, 1986
64. Sadé J: Pathogenesis of attic cholesteatoma. J Roy Soc Med 71: 716–732, 1978
65. Buckingham RA: The clinical appearance and natural history of cholesteatoma. In: *Cholesteatoma and Mastoid Surgery*. Sadé J (ed). Amsterdam: Kugler Publications 1982
66. Gigi-Leitner O, Geiger B, Levy R, Czernobilsky B: Cytokeratin expression in squamous metaplasia of the human uterine cervix. Differentiation 31: 191–205, 1986
67. Smedts F, Ramaekers F, Robben H, Pruszczynski M, Van Muijen G, Lane B, Leigh I, Vooijs P: Changing patterns of keratin expression during progression of cervical intraepithelial neoplasia. Am J Pathol 136: 657–668, 1990
68. Michaels L (ed): *Ear, Nose and Throat Histopathology*. Berlin: Springer Verlag 1987
69. Sando I, Suehiro S, Wood RP: Congenital anomalies of the external and middle ear. In: *Pediatric Otolaryngology*. Vol. I. Bluestone CD, Stool SE, Arjona SK (eds). Philadelphia: WB Saunders Co. 1983

CONGENITAL AURAL ATRESIA
Patient selection and surgical management

ROBERT A. JAHRSDOERFER

Department of Otolaryngology – Head and Neck Surgery, University of Texas Medical School, Houston, TX 77030, USA

Introduction

The surgical repair of congenital aural atresia is a formidable task and should be undertaken only by an experienced ear surgeon. It is not an operation for the novice. The operation is difficult and in the hands of an inexperienced surgeon there is a very real chance of injuring the patient.

Over 700 patients with a congenital ear malformation have been evaluated by the author. Over 350 patients have been operated upon. From these statistics, it can be appreciated that only one half of those patients with atresia ever come to surgery. In syndromic patients, *i.e.*, those with Treacher Collins syndrome or hemifacial microsomia, the percentage is even less, about 25%.

Preoperative evaluation

The preoperative evaluation will determine if the patient is a candidate for surgery. The evaluation routinely includes behavioral audiometry, auditory brainstem response testing, and high resolution CT imaging of the temporal bone. CT imaging is the single most important study done preoperatively. It is performed in the 30° axial and 105° coronal views and yields information that can be graded.

Computed tomography permits a careful selection of patients in whom successful surgery is usually predictable. It also allows 'impossible' cases to be avoided. Absolute indications for surgery in patients with congenital aural atresia include normal cochlear function and an intact inner ear on CT scanning. Magnetic resonance studies are of little use insofar as bone is not imaged.

Unilateral atresia is operated routinely. The only distinction made between unilateral and bilateral atresia is that in bilateral cases stringent criteria are sometimes relaxed to allow at least one ear to be operated.

It is important to tell the patient, or parents, that other options are available. These include: (1) a bone conducting hearing aid, (2) an implantable bone conducting device, (3) an air conduction hearing aid if a meatal pit is present, and (4) the surgical creation of an ear canal only to accommodate an ear level hearing aid in an otherwise non-surgical candidate.

While there still is controversy over who operates first, the plastic surgeon or the ear surgeon, this is now perceived as a non-issue. In every patient with grade III microtia, reconstruction of the auricle should precede atresia repair. The author has never seen a cosmetically acceptable external ear when atresia surgery was done first. Atresia repair may be performed anytime after the second stage of microtia repair (transposition of the lobule). The surgery should be planned jointly by the plastic

Middle Ear Structure, Organogenesis and Congenital Defects, pp. 81–83
edited by B. Ars and P. van Cauwenberge
©*1991 Kugler Publications, Amsterdam, New York*

surgeon and ear surgeon who will then combine their best talents for the good of the patient.

Surgical technique

All operations are done under general anesthesia. The patient is placed in a supine position with the involved ear up. Only a small swath of hair measuring about one half inch needs to be shaved about the ear. A postauricular incision is made routinely. The ear is reflected anteriorly and the periosteum and soft tissue are elevated off the lateral surface of the mastoid bone. Assuming there is complete atresia, the surgeon looks for a tympanic bone remnant as this will point the way to the middle ear. If one is not found, an alternate landmark is the cribriform area. The site of the temporomandibular joint is noted. Drilling is begun in the cribriform area staying high and hugging the tegmen. This direction will best avoid a displaced facial nerve. Air cell tracts are followed medially. It is important to stay out of the mastoid. As drilling progresses, an anterior bony canal wall is created between the new ear canal and the glenoid fossa. At a variable depth, most often 1.5 cm, the body of the incus is encountered. This is the first landmark identified. Confirmation is made by gentle palpation. Although the malformed ossicular chain is usually fixed to the atretic plate at the level of the malleus neck, the fused incus/malleus complex in the attic will be mobile on gentle palpation.

Drilling is continued to further delineate the ossicular chain. It is important to know that the malleus handle is usually absent. There often is a dense periosteal band that runs from the malformed malleus neck to the temporomandibular joint passing through a defect in the bony wall separating the joint from the middle ear. This band may be confused with an aberrant facial nerve and should be resected only after the facial nerve has been positively identified. Drilling is continued to gain room peripherally at the level of the middle ear. This technique centers the ossicular mass in the approximate middle of the new tympanic membrane. Once exposure of the middle ear is improved, the stapes is assessed, the mobility of the footplate is confirmed, and the position of the facial nerve is noted. It is not unusual for the facial nerve to be naked in its course through the middle ear. The stapes is often smaller than normal and the long arm of the incus is commonly crooked and foreshortened. All of these observations are of little significance clinically as long as the ossicular chain is otherwise intact and moves as a unit.

Temporalis fascia is used to create a new tympanic membrane. The edges of the fascia graft are reflected onto the newly drilled bony external ear canal for a short distance only – about 2 mm. A thin split thickness skin graft is harvested from the meatal aspect of the ipsilateral upper arm. This is sized, notched, and positioned in the ear canal to line the bare bone. The medial notched edges of the skin graft are reflected onto the fascia graft tympanic membrane. A Silastic button is placed over the reflected skin edges to secure them in place and to prevent blunting of the anterior and inferior sulci. Merocel is strategically placed in the bony ear canal and then hydrated.

A new meatus is constructed by incising an elliptical core of skin and soft tissue in the proper anatomical location. After the external ear has been tacked in position, the edges of the skin graft are identified, brought laterally, and sutured to the skin of the new meatus. Additional packing is placed to stabilize the lateral portion of the newly created ear canal.

The surgical procedure usually takes five hours and the child remains in the hospital overnight. The following day the mastoid dressing is removed and the child is discharged. Scarlet red dressing is used over the skin graft donor site. The gauze covering this area is removed (excluding the scarlet red dressing) on postoperative day one and the donor site is left uncovered to the air. The scarlet red dressing will slough in approximately ten to 14 days, revealing healthy pink skin beneath.

Postoperative care

All packing and sutures are removed one week postoperatively. A steroid/antibiotic ear drop preparation is used for five days after which nothing is placed in the ear. The patient returns four weeks postoperatively at which time the skin graft will have desquamated and there will be a large crust in the ear canal. This is gently removed revealing healthy skin lining the new ear canal and surface of the tympanic membrane. At this junction any redundant skin folds may be sharply excised. Behavioral audiometry is performed, and assuming a good result, the speech reception threshold will be between 15–25 dB. This can be achieved in 70–75% of patients. The patient is then discharged from care to return every six to 12 months for routine cleaning of the external ear canal. It is important to remember that although the ear canal skin is healthy and viable, it lacks memory and will not migrate as skin does in normal ear canals. This means that crusts will form, much like in a mastoid bowl, and must be mechanically cleaned at periodic intervals.

No restrictions are placed on the patient. He or she is allowed to swim with the only condition being the mandated use of one or two drops of an alcohol/boric acid ear preparation after each outing.

Postoperative stenosis of the meatus is a possible complication. This is seen most often when there is only soft tissue in that area. If there is conchal cartilage, stenosis does not usually occur as the cartilage maintains the size of the meatus. Although stents and molds are not used, it may be necessary to make the meatal opening larger than normal if cartilage is not present. A meatal cartilaginous ring may be constructed and inserted at the time of atresia surgery, or may be prepared and placed earlier by the plastic surgeon at the time of microtia repair.

High frequency sensorineural hearing loss will occur in 10% of patients despite pure tone thresholds being normal or near normal. While the risk of facial nerve injury is always present, this seldom occurs in the hands of an experienced operator.

CONSIDERATIONS ON THE SURGICAL TREATMENT OF CONGENITAL EAR ATRESIA

J. MARQUET and F. DECLAU

Department of Otorhinolaryngology (Head: Prof Dr J Marquet), University of Antwerp, Wilrijk, Belgium

Introduction

As extensively discussed in our report on congenital middle ear malformations at the Belgian ENT Society in 1988[1], the two main questions to be answered are: how to prevent middle ear malformations, and how to cure them surgically.

The main goal in the treatment of congenital middle ear pathology is to provide a serviceable improvement of the hearing as well as to help people who have psychological problems due to the cosmetic appearance of their malformation.

As quoted by Rapin and Ruben[2], the clinicians treating such children must balance the benefits expected from the procedure they are offering against the possible complications.

Nevertheless, faced with the tremendous problems related to this type of surgery, and regarding its functional and cosmetic aspects, our first duty at the end of the twentieth century is to obtain a better knowledge of prevention of these abnormalities, by improved studies in embryology, genetics or teratology.

Medical genetics

The main developmental abnormalities may be genetically or purely environmentally induced.

Three types of genetic anomalies have been identified: single mutant genes, chromosomal abnormalities and abnormalities due to multifactorial inheritance.

The single mutant genes type concentrates on the associated patterns of Mendelian inheritance: autosomal dominant, autosomal recessive and X- or Y-linked. Distinction between these patterns is essential for determining the recurrence risks (Table 1).

Chromosomal abnormalities can be identified by staining methods for metameric chromosomes.

Multifactorial inheritance is determined by multiple genetic and non-genetic factors, each making a relatively small contribution to the phenotype.

These three patterns are not always easy to distinguish. Common problems in dealing with Mendelian inheritance are the presence of reduced penetrance, new mutations and consanguinity.

In multifactorial inheritance a variety of models can be constructed to fit the empirical data. Everything depends on how much of the variation is due to segregating genes and how much to environmental factors. Although there is a continuous distribution in multifactorial inheritance, usually a developmental threshold is defined by

Middle Ear Structure, Organogenesis and Congenital Defects, pp. 85–98
edited by B. Ars and P. van Cauwenberge
©*1991 Kugler Publications, Amsterdam, New York*

TABLE 1. Recurrence risks caused by single mutant gene

	One parent affected % risk in in each child	Parents unaffected % risk in sibs	Parents unaffected % risk sibs
Autosomal recessive	0	25	25
Autosomal dominant	50	0	0
X-linked recessive	0	0	50
			(assuming mother is carrier)

separating it into two discontinuous segments: with and without the malformation.

Until now, multifactorial inheritance has not been identified among the causes of deafness. According to Jaffe, the most likely explanation is that family studies have not been designed to distinguish between multifactorial inheritance and single mutant genes as the cause of deafness.

The phenomenon of sporadic cases with normal chromosomes constitutes a great problem in genetic counseling. It may be interpreted in various ways:
1. Purely environmentally induced.
2. New mutation of an autosomal dominant trait.
3. Autosomal recessive disorder.
4. Reduced penetrance in an autosomal dominant trait.
5. X-linked disorder in a male proband in whom the mother is carrier.
6. Multifactorial inheritance with low recurrence rate.

In view of the family history and the diagnosis, the most appropriate possibility must be chosen cautiously.

It is beyond doubt that genetic counseling as well as environmental protection becomes essential in order to prevent malformations for the coming decades.

Surgical treatment

Three main problems are to be taken into account when surgery is considered.

a. The surgical approaches to the middle ear cleft and the remaining ossicles: the classical approach, by which a large antro-attico-mastoidectomy is created, and the less popular technique applied by us, which consists of an approach similar to the combined approach tympanoplasty technique, in which a new posterior wall is created (Fig. 1)

b. The cosmetic aspect in congenital middle ear surgery.

c. The new techniques using implantable auditive prosthetic materials.

From the outset, *i.e.*, from the last decades of the past century when Kiesselbach[3] was credited in 1883 for performing the first deep operation on a child with congenital atresia, the leading principle for each proposed surgical technique has always and solely been only related to the opening of the atretic plate and the creation in some way of a new sound-conducting canal or bypass towards the middle ear cleft. Middle

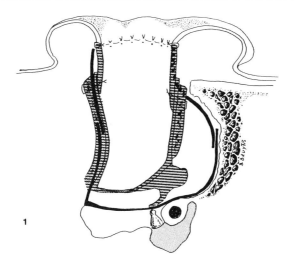

Fig. 1.

ear surgical approaches were proposed and applied, without real knowledge of embryology and patho-anatomy relating to maldevelopments of the middle ear. In 1978[4] Jahrsdoerfer published an excellent overview of the evolution of this surgery over the past 50 years: in 1930 the usual surgical technique consisted of making a very small opening in the atretic plate before covering this area with a skin graft, or even, as reported by the same authors, creating a patent Eustachian tube as a way of providing a bypass for sound to the atretic ear[5]. In the same period, discussion about the preservation of malleus and incus arose.

Most of the authors such as Colver, Pattee, Ombredanne, Livingstone advocated the removal of these ossicles because of their functional uselessness in the absence of a tympanic membrane, or even considered them as obstacles to the normal mobility of the stapes.

Controversy about the approach to the atretic middle ear led to different techniques of meatoplasty: as small as possible and covered with a split-thickness skin graft (Pattee) or on the contrary, as large as possible and covered with a full-thickness skin graft (Ombredanne). According to Wullstein and Zöllner, the main principles of tympanoplasty were transferred to congenital ear surgery: these involved a large opening of the bony plate in association with large mastoidectomies.

In this type of surgery, Ombredanne reported the first results in 1949 on the application of the fenestration technique in cases where the stapes was not functional. Since then, the general rules have not changed very much. Up to now the creation of large cavities, covered by grafting material using skin or fascia temporalis, is routinely applied. Enthusiastically faced with the present state of art in functional surgery of deafness and its success in other types of surgery, many authors have transferred their modern tympanoplasty techniques to surgery for congenital middle ear malformations.

Regardless of the grafting material used: skin grafts, fascia grafts, allogenous tissue or preserved tympanomeatal allografts, the main controversy between these techniques does not essentially lie in a different philosophy. The main issue is indeed what

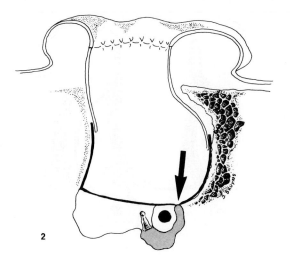

Fig. 2.

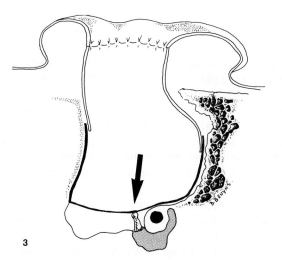

Fig. 3.

Belluci, Roulleau, Derlacki and many others are concerned about: can an atretic plate be widened sufficiently to accommodate a full-size tympano-meatal allograft?

In our 25 years experience, the correct use of tympano-ossicular or tympano-meatal allografts in congenital middle ear surgery[6-8], has proved that the long-term results are excellent and even superior to all other techniques. We may also assert that in congenital middle ear surgery an anatomical restoration of the middle ear, as obtained by the allograft techniques, gives the greatest guarantees in congenital middle ear surgery.

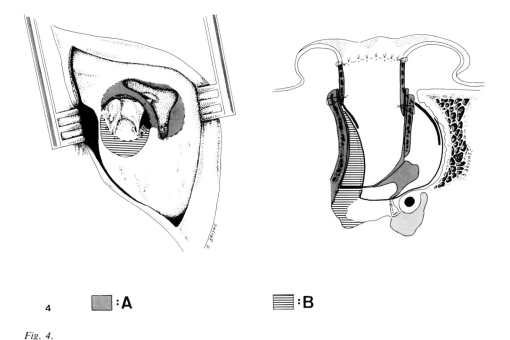

4   ▨ :A   ▤ :B

Fig. 4.

Large cavities versus meatoplasty techniques

Large cavities of classical techniques are based on the following principles: the cavity shall be created as large as possible in order to avoid postoperative stenosis, which is absolutely correct when tympano-meatal allografts are not used.

The sound transmission system is commonly restored by using the fenestration technique (Fig. 2) or by a Wullstein type III (Fig. 3). The newly created cavity must therefore be centered either on the external semicircular canal or on the head of the stapes: for this reason, the hypotympanum is never enlarged.

It is always disregarded and represents in all the classical procedures the inferior limit for drilling out the atretic plate. In our technique of meatoplasty, where the implantation of a deep meatal allograft cuff is indispensable for avoiding stenosis, and where a new posterior wall is created, the enlargement of the hypotympanum is an absolute prerequisite, since a new bony annulus must be sculptured for the embedding of the implanted fibro-cartilaginous annulus of the graft (Fig. 4). Hence, a better and appropriate knowledge of this area allows us to displace the drilled-out cavity inferiorly, to the extent that in relation to the ossicles and the otic capsule, the anatomical repositioning of a normally sized tympanic membrane becomes possible. So far, we may summarize that the difference between these two surgical concepts lies in the level of approach to the otic capsule, as shown in Fig. 5a and b. The use of fascia seems to us not appropriate for this technique because of the risk of stenosis.

Of course, one has to pay particular attention to the anatomy of this area and to the possible abnormal routes of the facial nerve in this inferior area of atretic ears, according to the anatomo-surgical classification in type I and II[9,10].

We may conclude that the main features of our surgical technique are based on

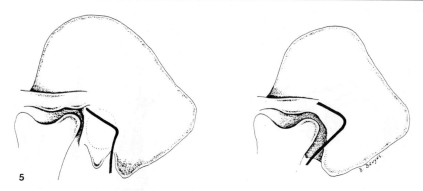

5

Fig. 5.

the use of a tympano-meatal or monobloc allograft and we regard congenital aural atresia as one of the main indications for its use[11]. In a one-stage procedure, it is possible to produce a safe anatomical reconstruction of the external auditory canal, valuable functional hearing improvement and very acceptable cosmetic appearance.

Complications

In spite of the fact that this type of surgery is generally practised on healthy and even noninfected ears, the encountered complications to be discussed are the same as in normal middle ear surgery: by definition, the postoperative complications are postoperative states that do not meet the expected goal of the surgical procedure as regards healing, anatomy, or function[12].

Infection

Since the main common infectious complication is usually bacterial, this can affect any operated ear. Contamination of a surgically treated congenital middle ear cleft may arise from the nasopharynx or from the newly created external ear canal. While immediate postoperative infections are extremely rare, delayed infectious complications may occur, and this more frequently when a large cavity has been created, in other words, when the classical procedure has been used. In the allograft technique this type of complication is extremely rare, because a new tympanic barrier between the canal skin and the middle ear mucosal layer is anatomically correctly replaced. The most common causative agents are *Streptococcus pyogenes*, *Staphylococcus aureus*, *Pseudomonas aeruginosa* and *Candida albicans*.

Granuloma

A nonsuppurative *granulomatous* covering of the middle ear and the mastoid cavity, represents one of the most frequently encountered postoperative complications when large cavities have been made (Fig. 6a). Occasionally, in the allograft technique, when the skin does not grow over the graft, the tympanic membrane and the depth of the newly created canal are covered by a granulomatous layer (Fig. 6b). A

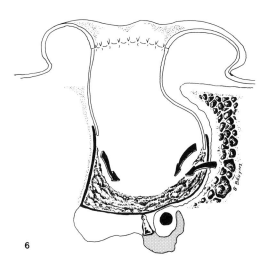

Fig. 6.

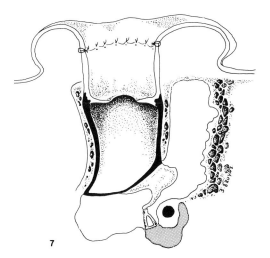

Fig. 7.

squamo-mucosal or *squamo-granulomatous* interface then remains. Formation of a stenotic ring may lead to a real stenotic membrane (Fig. 7). This complication, which can also appear in a great number of newly created large cavities, has been observed in only 14% of our cases, making this the most frequent complication in the allograft technique.

Absence of squamous epithelial migration

The absence of squamous epithelial migration is associated with the same pathological phenomenon as that responsible for the previously mentioned complication.

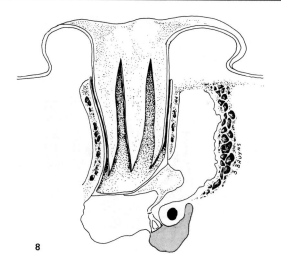

Fig. 8.

The recent and prominent studies of Proops *et al.*[13] in the field of tissue culture of migratory skin of the external ear, and of Broekaert[14] in the study of cytokeratin, have given the most plausible explanation of this problem. These authors have indeed proven that extraconchal skin colonies grew with the formation of a cuff, which allowed them to fuse with each other. Nevertheless, as migratory skin and cholesteatoma explants matured, while initially resembling normal skin, they never grew as large and did not conflue. After three weeks, colony growth in normal skin appeared to slow down. On the contrary, colonies of migratory skin and cholesteatoma explants exhibited mass movement. After about 21 days in culture the colonies were seen to exhibit a polarity: the cells all became elongated in the same axis. Once mass movement was established, the colonies tended to continue moving in their chosen directions.

Summarizing, everything acted as if the genuine migration pattern of intraconchal or intrameatal skin was much more active and similarly oriented along an axis in contrast with the migration pattern of extraconchal skin.

Clinically, we have observed this phenomenon for years: in atresia type I for instance, when remnants of meatal or canal skin exist and they are stripped and replaced, covering even partially the cuff of the graft, no problems of skin migration occur (Fig. 8). On the contrary, like in the majority of the atresia type II cases, when only a full extraconchal skin flap can be used to cover the graft, migration seems to be delayed or even blocked and granulation will appear in the depth of the canal.

In unilateral cases, it has also been proven that free skin grafts taken from the drum or in the external ear canal of the normal ear keep their original migration patterns. This will guarantee a complete covering of drum and canal walls, better than a split-thickness skin graft.

Cholesteatoma

In the long run, cholesteatoma or, more frequently, epithelial debris can be found in large cavities because of a lack of self-cleaning capacities. Here also, the advantage of the use of tympano-meatal allografts lies in the fact that in a new canal self-cleaning properties are restored.

Later displacement

The lateral displacement of the newly implanted drum may be confused with the above reported stenotic membrane. The diagnosis may sometimes be difficult by simple otoscopic examination: while in the stenotic membrane a space between the non-epithelialized tympanic membrane and the skin membrane does exist, in the lateral displacement the epithelialized membrane as a whole moves laterally and disjunction with the ossicles appears.

In a second stage procedure, the replacement of such a laterally displaced tympanic membrane in the depth of the canal is indispensable.

Sero-mucous otitis

As in other types of middle ear surgery, a new conductive hearing loss may appear due to mucosal pathology with hyperplasia of goblet cells and loss of cilia function.

Stenosis and osteolysis

Recurrent bony growth resulting in a secondary stenosis of the newly created external auditory canal is the most feared complication in the techniques where the opening into the middle ear is made as small as possible regardless whether it is covered by a split-thickness skin graft or by a fascia graft. This complication has led the majority of the authors to advocate the creation of very large openings. When a tympano-meatal allograft is used, this complication may be considered as inexistent. Histological studies have indeed proven that behind the implanted meatal graft acting as periosteum, a true neo-cortical bony layer is formed.

Osteolysis may be considered as an exceptional complication, except of course when infection is involved.

Ossicular ankylosis

Ankylosis or reankylosis of the original or implanted ossicles seem to be very rare in our experience. Nevertheless, it should be mentioned that great risk for reankylosis exists when the surgical field and the created middle ear cleft is not properly and regularly cleaned from bone dust or bone debris during surgery.

Functional complications

The study of vestibular and audiological complications of operated ears is essential in the postoperative evaluation: since fenestration is not commonly used anymore in congenital ear surgery, damage to the vestibular organs is very exceptional. No cases have been reported in our series.

Acoustic trauma

Accidental injury to the labyrinth may be caused by too high sound energy. This may happen with any kind of burr, but especially with cutting burrs that make contact with ossicles which are still connected with the inner ear. Noise produced by such drilling is between 160 and 200 dB[15]. In congenital malformations, the risk of acoustic trauma is high if no special care is taken during surgery, because of the frequent occurrence of a mobile stapes connected with a fixed incus or more frequently with a malleus fixed at the atretic plate. In such situations, the use of curettes or even better, of laser, is the ideal solution.

Inner ear damage

The application of techniques such as stapedectomies and stapedotomies or as more recently introduced by Plester[16], trepanation of the labyrinth seems to us very controversial in this type of surgery. It should only be advocated in isolated malformations with normal tympanic membrane and after CT examination in order to exclude any associated inner ear malformation.

No risk of sensorineural hearing loss may be incurred in surgery on already handicapped patients.

Audiological complications have to be distinguished into two groups: a postoperative functional state, which is not in agreement with the expected goal of surgery, can occur because of a failure to restore the sound transmission system of the middle ear or because of one of the above mentioned complications; the second group concerns postoperative states in which a new and unexpected neurosensorial loss has taken place.

Facial nerve injury

In none of our operated cases was facial nerve paralysis observed. With a better understanding of the developmental anatomy of atresia, this serious complication might not occur.

Cosmetic surgery

The new external auditory canal must be rebuilt in functional continuity with the middle ear cavity and ossicular chain. The canal must be reconstituted before any cosmetic surgery is carried out: this may be simultaneously or in a second stage, but must never be done before the functional stage. Plastic surgery of the pinna is only acceptable if it is centered on the new meatus and the otic capsule. This is an advantage for our allograft meatoplasty technique, since it is based on the reconstitution of normal anatomical landmarks.

Auricular reconstruction has been a challenge as early as 600 B.C. In 1830 total reconstruction was considered as impracticable, but since 1890 many different techniques have been tried out, using all kinds of frames in different materials. Often surgery had to be done over and over again, before any results were achieved.

However, the retention of a prosthesis has often been a problem. One method is the incorporation of the auricular prosthesis as a part of eyeglasses; adhesive or double-sided adhesive tape is often used for attachment, but may cause adverse skin reactions, or discoloration. The method of retaining the prosthesis by bone-anchored titanium implants eliminates these drawbacks. The successful long-term use of bone-anchored dental bridges, as described by Adell *et al.* in 1981[17], introduced this new method to retain prostheses.

In 1977 the first titanium implants in the temporal bone were performed and the first bone-anchored hearing aid was installed[18].

The hearing aid was anchored directly in bone with a skin penetrating titanium device as described by Tjellström in 1985[19]. The favorable clinical results experienced at the ENT-Department in Göteborg have led to a clinical routine procedure to anchor, not only hearing aids, but also to utilize the method of skin penetrating titanium devices for the attachment of prostheses to restore the external ear and other craniofacial defects.

Implant surgery

The idea to develop an implantable hearing aid originated from the many disadvantages of the conventional hearing aid, such as acoustic feed-back, tight earmold and the cosmetic appearance of wearing a prosthesis.

Some patients who need a hearing aid are unable to use an air conduction hearing aid which transmits sound via the external ear canal. These patients may benefit from a conventional bone conduction hearing aid. The bone conductor is applied by a steel spring or on the temples of a pair of glasses, over the mastoid process, and the sound is transmitted via the soft tissues and the bone to the cochlea. The apparance is not cosmetically satisfactory and the force needed to apply the transducer often causes discomfort to the patient.

In the seventies, several researchers started producing devices aiming at the implantable hearing aid, and recently the implantable hearing aid, which has reached a remarkable development. In this short overview we shall describe the Brånemark hearing aid, first introduced in 1977, the implantable devices of Hough and the middle ear implant of Suzuki, both introduced in humans in 1984.

The bone-anchored hearing aid (BAHA) introduced by Brånemark, Tjellström et al.

Based on the experience with dental implants – a report on more than 3,000 implants in the jaws had been published[17] – the idea of inserting titanium implants in the temporal bone for fixation of a hearing aid by bone conduction was raised. Another clinical application of these implants in the temporal bone is the fixation of an auricular prosthesis. Since 1977, several hundreds of titanium implants have been inserted into the temporal bone in humans, with excellent results.

The BAHA is characterized by a single housing construction. The transducer piston of the BAHA is directly connected to the titanium screw by a low-profile coupling arrangement, through skin penetration. Since 1977 there have been first-

and second-generation hearing aids, and several principles for realizing the single housing apparatus have been tested.

Implantable bone conduction hearing device: audiant bone conductor (ABC), introduced by Hough et al.

The ABC is composed of an internal and external device. The internal implantable part consists of a small rare earth magnet (samarium cobalt) housed in a titanium disk attached to an orthopedic screw.

The magnet is sealed with medical grade silicone. By the use of specially designed tapping instruments, this screw-magnet assembly is implanted under local anesthesia in the sinodural angle of the skull. This magnet is caused to vibrate by electromagnetic fields produced by the external device. The external device is composed of a sound processor consisting of a microphone and an electronic package with amplifying circuitry, battery power supply, and controls. This is connected to an inductive coil with a magnetic core of SmCO5.

The magnetic core of the coil holds the device on the skin directly over the implanted magnet-screw assembly, thus allowing transcutaneous transfer of energy. The sound signal is then conducted by bone vibrations directly to the inner ear.

There have been three generations of ABC sound processors. The last generation processor, the 3-V body unit, has become much smaller, and in addition, asks much less of the battery.

Miniaturization is still foreseeable, and a functional behind-the-ear-unit has recently been introduced.

Middle ear implant introduced by Suzuki et al. – principle and reconstruction

Two types of middle ear implant (MEI) in connection with an artificial middle ear project, have been developed. One is a totally implantable hearing aid, the other a partially implantable device. The main difference between the MEI and the conventional hearing aid lies in energy transmission to the stapes. The implant consists of a microphone (input transducer), an amplifier, a battery and a ceramic vibrator (output transducer).

One tip of the ceramic vibrator has an apatite attachment to the stapes, while the other has an apatite base to the bone. The vibrator, consisting of piezoelectric ceramic, vibrates with voltage changes, and the vibration follows electrical signals very faithfully. Sounds are transduced to electrical signals by the microphone. The electrical signals are amplified and transduced by the ceramic vibrator to the mechanical vibration of the stapes.

In the conventional hearing aid, signal energy is transduced to vibration of air in the external auditory canal and transmitted to the inner ear through the middle ear. In the conventional bone conduction hearing aids, signal energy is transmitted directly to the inner ear by vibration of the skull, where energy consumption should be much greater compared with the MEI.

In the partially implantable MEI an internal induction coil and a vibrator are constructed as implantable components. The external components are a microphone, an amplifier, a battery and an external induction coil. Incoming sounds are converted into electrical signals by the microphone, and these are amplified and transmitted from the external to the internal coil. The vibrator converts the electrical signals into the mechanical vibration of the stapes and transmits it to the inner ear. In the totally implantable device, the microphone, amplifier, a battery and the vibrator are implanted. As a power supply, two types of battery are prepared; they work for at least three years *in vivo*.

Conclusion

However, except in ear agenesis from type I the long-term listing of the functional results appears rather disappointing. The characteristics of this type are extensively discussed elsewhere[1].

The audiological prognosis must therefore depend on the involved type I or II. In type I, the atresia is only the consequence of abnormal development of the tympanic ring. The facial nerve always follows its normal topography.

The middle ear anomalies of the ossicular chain are minimal and only a fibrotic or osteotic occlusion of the medial two-thirds of the external canal exists. In this type, the characteristic space and the distance between the posterior wall of the glenoid cavity and the anterior part of the mastoid not only always exist but are generally constant and normal. On the contrary, in type II atresia the abnormal development of middle ear structures is considerably worse. These cases are recognized by the absence of the characteristic space between the posterior wall of the glenoid cavity and the anterior part of the mastoid, which is situated in the immediate neighborhood of the mandibular articulation. The topography of the facial nerve is always abnormal. Everything works as if the space corresponding to the os tympanicum is missing. This topographical analysis must be done pre-operatively by radiological evaluation. More recently, this concept of classification into these two types has also been advocated by De La Cruz *et al.*[20] and Cremers *et al.*[21].

These disappointing results in type II atresia are commonly due to delayed and permanent discharging cavities, delayed stenosis of the newly created auditory canal.

Nevertheless, this surgery of middle ear atresia must certainly not be abandoned, with the understanding that it may never fall into the hands of occasional and untrained ear surgeons; on the contrary, it should be the subject for further study and research.

Also, research on implantable cosmetic as well as hearing aids prosthetic material should be developed and improved.

References

1. Marquet JF, Declau F, De Cock M, De Paep K, Appel B, Moeneclaey L: Congenital middle ear malformations. Acta ORL Belg 42(2): 23–302, 1988
2. Ruben RJ, Rapin I: Plasticity of the developing auditory system. Ann Otol Rhinol Laryngol 89: 303–311, 1980
3. Kiesselbach W: Ersuch zur Anlegung eines ausseren Gehörganges bei angeborener Missbildung beider Ohrmuschel mit Fehlen der ausseren Gehörgange. Arch Ohrenheilk Leipz 19: 127–131, 1982
4. Jahrsdoefer RA: Congenital malformations of the ear. Analysis of 94 operations. Ann Otol Rhinol Laryngol 89: 348–352, 1980

5. Randall BA: Remarks in: Congenital bilateral microtia with total osseous atresia of the external auditory canals, operation and report of cases, by Page JR. Trans Am Otol Soc 13: 376–390, 1914
6. Lenz W: Das Thalidomid Syndrom. Fortschr Med 81: 148, 1963
7. Marquet JF: Homogreffes tympano-malléaires dans le traitement chirurgical des agénésies d'oreilles. CR Congrès Soc ORL Franç 1969
8. Marquet JF: Allografts and congenital aural atresia. Adv Otol Rhinol Laryngol 40: 21, 1987
9. Marquet JF: Congenital malformations and middle ear surgery. J Roy Soc Med 74: 119–128, 1981
10. Marquet JF: Congenital conductive deafness. In: Maran GD, Stell PM (eds): *Clinical Otolaryngology*, pp 501–513. Oxford: Blackwell Scientific 1979
11. Marquet JF: Homografts in tympanoplasty and other forms of middle ear surgery. In: *Operative Surgery*. London: Butterworth 1989
12. Marquet JF: A classification of operative procedures and their complications. Complications in Otolaryngology Head and Neck Surgery. In: Wiet R, Caus JB (eds): *Ear and Skull Base*, pp 1–7, 1986
13. Proops DW, Hawke WM, Parkinson EK: Tissue culture of migratory skin of the external ear and cholesteatoma: a new research tool. J Otolaryngol 13(2): 63–69, 1984
14. Broekaert D, Coucke P, Reyniers P, Marquet J: Keratinization of middle ear cholesteatomas. A histochemical study of epidermal transglutaminase substrates. Eur Arch Otolaryngol 247: 318–322, 1990
15. Helms J: J Laryngol Otol 90: 1143–1149, 1976
16. Plester D: Congenital middle ear pathology (abstract). Acta ORL Belg 9: 182, 1971
17. Adell R, Lekholm U, Rockler B, Brånemark PI: A 15 year study of osseointegrated implants in the treatment of the edentulous jaw. Int J Oral Surg 10: 387, 1982
18. Tjellström A, Yountchev E, Lindström J, Brånemark PI: Five years experience with bone-anchored auricular prostheses. Otolaryngol Head Neck Surg 93: 366–772, 1985
19. Tjellström A, Lindström J, Hallen O, Albrektsson T, Brånemark PI: Osseointegrated titanium implants in the temporal bone. Am J Otol 2: 304–310, 1981
20. De La Cruz A, Linthicum FH, Luxford WM: Congenital atresia of the external auditory canal. Laryngoscope 95: 421–427, 1985
21. Cremers CWRS, Marres EH: An additional classification for congenital aural atresia. Its impact on the predictability of surgical results. Acta ORL Belg 41: 4, 1987

Authors index